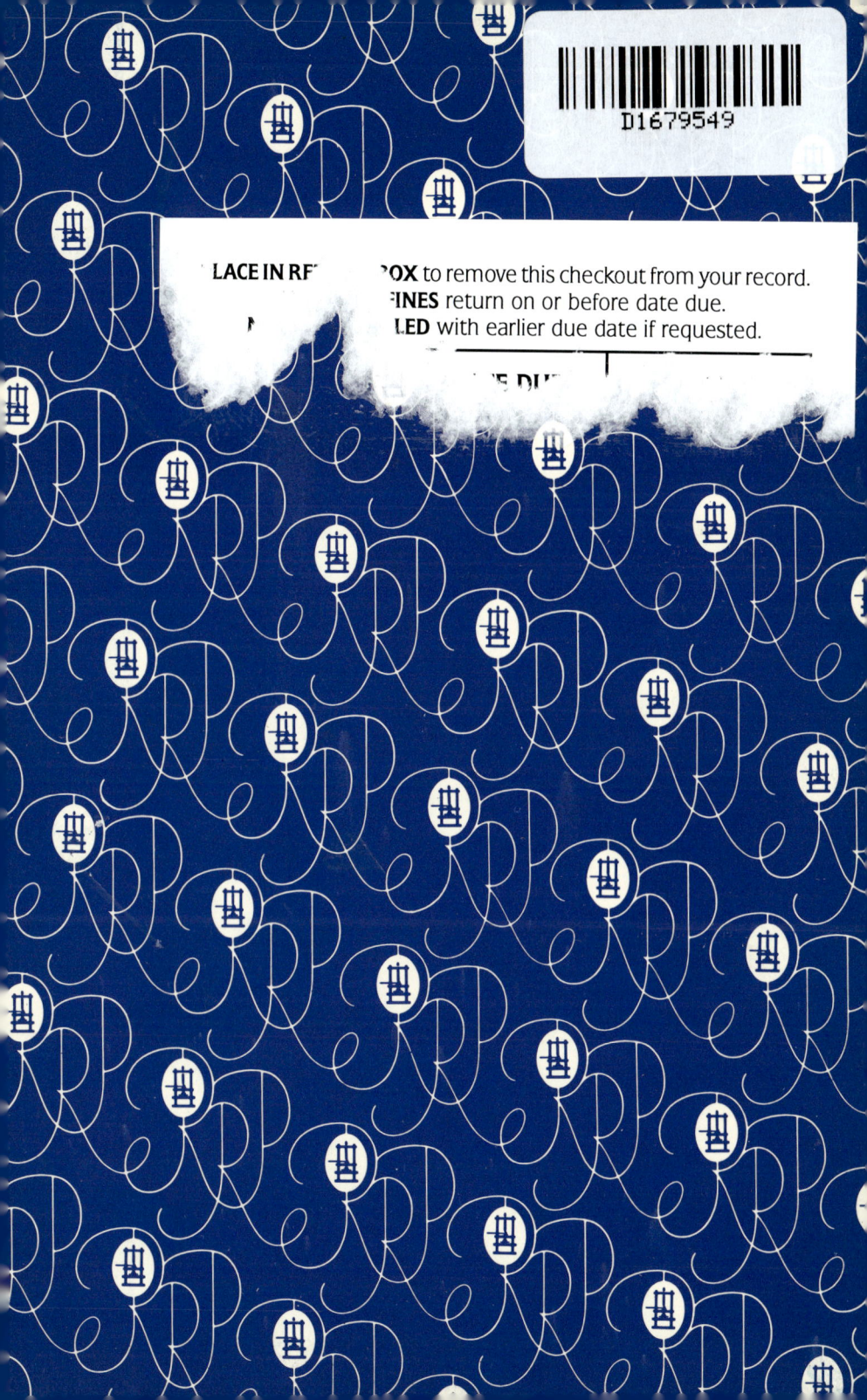

YOUR FUTURE IN VETERINARY MEDICINE

YOUR FUTURE IN VETERINARY MEDICINE

Wayne H. Riser, D.V.M., M.S.,
Dr.med.vet., M.A. (Hon.)

RICHARDS ROSEN PRESS, INC.
New York, New York 10010

SF
779.5
.R56
1982
c.2

Published in 1970, 1977, 1982 by Richards Rosen Press, Inc.
29 East 21st Street, New York City, New York 10010

Revised Edition 1982
Copyright 1970, 1977 by Wayne H. Riser

All rights reserved. No part of this book may be produced
in any form without permission in writing from
the publisher, except by a reviewer.

Library of Congress Cataloging in Publication Data

Riser, Wayne H
  Your future in veterinary medicine.

  Bibliography: p.
  1. Veterinary medicine—Vocational guidance.
I. Title. [DNLM: 1. Veterinary medicine—Juvenile
literature. SF744 R595y]
SF779.5.R56 1978   636.089'069   77-2695
ISBN 0-8239-0400-8

Manufactured in the United States of America

About the Author

DR. WAYNE H. RISER received his D.V.M. and M.S. in pathology from Iowa State University, a doctorate in pathology from the University of Bern and a M.A. (Hon.) from the University of Pennsylvania. He is a Diplomate of the American College of Veterinary Pathology.

After leaving practice in 1960, Doctor Riser served at the Armed Forces of Pathology, Washington, D.C. and at the School of Veterinary Medicine, University of Pennsylvania, Philadelphia, Pa. where he is an Emeritus Professor of Pathology. He presently serves as an Adjunct Professor of Pathology at University of Florida, Gainesville, Florida.

Doctor Riser is the recipient of a number of awards: Gaines Veterinarian of the Year Award; Mark L. Morris Small Animal Award; Iowa State University Stange Award; Michigan State University Centennial Award; A.V.M.A. Practition-Research Award; and Charles L. Davis Journal Scholarship Award.

He is past president of the American Animal Hospital Association, American Society of Veterinary Radiologists, Mid-West Small Animal Association, American College of Veterinary Pathology and the World Small Animal Veterinary Association.

Preface to Revised Edition

Since this book was published in 1977, many scientific and personnel changes have taken place. We have made the necessary changes in pertinent facts and figures and revised the salary ranges upward or downward depending on current conditions. The figures used are the most recent available.

Contents

Preface	ix
Introduction	xi
I. The History of Veterinary Medicine	3
II. The Diseases of Animals	22
III. Qualifications	26
IV. Veterinary Education	34
V. Veterinarians in Practice	49
VI. Veterinarians in Federal Services	79
VII. Veterinarians in Teaching and Research	101
VIII. Veterinarians in the Armed Forces and Space Medicine	111
IX. Veterinarians in Commercial Enterprises	117
X. Veterinarians in Nutrition	121
XI. Opportunities in Veterinary Science	125
XII. Women in Veterinary Medicine	130
XIII. The Veterinarian's License to Practice and the Code of Ethics	132
XIV. Your Future in Veterinary Medicine	137
Appendix I. Colleges of Veterinary Medicine in America	139
Appendix II. Veterinary Associations	142
Appendix III. Bibliography	145

Preface

It is not possible to describe the activities of veterinary medicine in one volume, for the scope is too broad. If, however, your enthusiasm for the profession is aroused or heightened by my brief discussion of its many facets, my efforts have been worthwhile.

The author is also appreciative of the assistance and encouragement of Dr. H. H. Dukes, who, after a full career as a teacher and research worker in veterinary medicine, is now donating his time to the recruitment of students for schools of veterinary medicine. Acknowledgment is also given to colleagues and professional friends who have given generously of their advice and encouragement.

> Dr. Wayne H. Riser, Professor Emeritus
> Department of Veterinary Pathology
> School of Veterinary Medicine
> University of Pennsylvania
> Philadelphia, Pennsylvania 19174

Introduction

The following is a letter typical of many received from high school students regarding Veterinary Medicine as a career.

Dear Sir:

I am a sophomore in high school and my counselor told me it would be all right to write you about becoming a veterinarian. I am very fond of animals, especially since I spent last summer on my uncle's farm.

Can you tell me more about what a veterinarian does and how to become one? Does it cost much to go to school? How long does it take? How does one go into practice and how much will one earn?

I would like to have your answer soon. Thank you for sending the information.

Sincerely,

This book will discuss Veterinary Medicine and the people in the profession. It may open the door to one of the most fascinating careers a young person can contemplate. I have spent my life in it, and my enthusiasm for it grows rather than diminishes. Since graduation from veterinary college some 40 years ago, I have seen the profession gain in stature and scope, and the potential for a young person entering the field today is tremendous.

Concern for animals is the primary requisite for this career, and the child who shows an early affinity and affection for animal pets possesses the most important single motivating factor for becoming a veterinarian. As this is expressed and he, or she, grows in experience with his own pets and other animals around him, especially if he is fortunate enough to live on a farm, his curiosity and his concern for their welfare leads to a desire to aid them when they are sick, to bind up their wounds, and to protect them from harm.

Most youngsters have experienced these feeling. Fostering this instinct leads to a growth of understanding of the fundamentals of life itself and the development of affection and compassion. I feel strongly that this phase of growing and the way in which it is nurtured contribute greatly to building good character in our young people.

From among these youngsters come those whose abiding interest and curiosity lead them to inquire into caring for animals as a life work. It is to them that this book is directed.

The majority of veterinarians are in either large-animal or small-animal practice, although many do both. They give animals care that is similar to the services rendered by physicans. A veterinarian must accordingly receive a similar medical education. It takes a minimum of three and usually four years of pre-veterinary college work and four years of veterinary medicine before a degree of D.V.M. or V.M.D. doctor of veterinary medicine, is earned. The graduate must then pass the state veterinary medical board examination in order to qualify for a license to practice.

There is no set internship requirement in veterinary medicine but most young doctors usually work for a year or more with an experienced veterinarian before they feel confident to establish their own practice or before they become associated in practice. Increasingly, as in human medicine, some veterinary graduates continue on in school for advanced training in a specialty. Medical science has progressed so rapidly and is becoming so complex that there is a growing need for graduate study.

Veterinary medicine, although an ancient calling, has developed more slowly than human medicine. But it is following the lead into more intense scientific research and, indeed, the two fields are benefiting more and more from a growing appreciation of their interdependence. The veterinarian is no longer just an old-fashioned "horse doctor." His skill has been refined and greatly enhanced by better scientific education, and today he no longer goes to the animal to treat it as often as he invites the owner to bring it to his well-equipped hospital or clinic where, with the necessary apparatus at hand, he can do a better job of diagnosis and treatment—just as physicians now do much more work in the clinics and hospitals than in the patient's home.

Also specialization has qualified veterinarians to provide service of much wider scope. They now contribute greatly to better nutrition, disease control, disease prevention, better public health, increased livestock production, dairy production, poultry production, medical research, and even Space Age exploration, as shown by the preparation and care of Enos, the chimpanzee, that made the first trip into space.

In the United States there are 35,500 active veterinarians, and there is an unfilled demand for many more. Sixteen new veterinary schools have been established since World War II making a total of 27 in the United States and 3 in

Canada. But our country needs still more veterinarians each year than these schools can graduate.

The field of veterinary medicine needs and welcomes qualified young people, and I hope that this book will serve to introduce you to it and to lead you to look into it further. Reading is a good way to learn about any field, and in the bibliography at the back of the book I refer you to some good autobiographies of veterinarians who tell of their very colorful careers, rich in accomplishment and the joy of doing the work they love.

Even better than reading, get to know some veterinarians. You will find them easy to approach, usually generous about giving their time to answer questions, and happy to tell you about their veterinary work and experiences. If they suggest that you are welcome to come into their hospital to watch them at work or to ride with them into the country on a call, accept readily and get a bit of the feel of what it is like to be a veterinarian. Such first-hand encounters often prove to be inspiring turning points that enrich both those who give and those who receive.

YOUR FUTURE IN VETERINARY MEDICINE

CHAPTER I

The History of Veterinary Medicine*

Ancient Civilization (2500 B.C. to 250 B.C.)

The dawn of veterinary medicine is recorded in ancient China, Babylonia, Egypt, and India in the earliest writings of civilization. In China, treatises on the diseases of horses and water buffalo were written as early as 2500 B.C. These describe the medicinal use of such substances as opium, aconite, croton, iron, arsenic, and sulfur. The Babylonian Code of Hammurabi (2200 B.C.) stipulated what medical fees were to be charged for the treatment of both man and beast, and set forth harsh penalties for malpractice as well as for the mistreatment of animals. In Egypt, the Ebers Papyrus (1550 B.C.) is the oldest complete medical book in existence. It contains 700 prescriptions, featuring such items as fly specks, crocodile dung, and whole mice. Ancient India (1800 B.C. to 1200 B.C.) has supplied the most concrete identification of the veterinary art. The leading veterinarian of that time was named Salihotra, and after

---

* Much of the material gathered for this chapter was abstracted from: J. F. Smithcors, "Evolution of the Veterinary Art," Kansas City, Veterinary Medical Publishing Company, 1957.

him all veterinarians were referred to as salihatrya. The present Indian term, Salutri, is a derivative of the ancient term.

In the Vedec period of India, the chief occupation was cattle raising. Prize bovines became closely associated with religion and the concept of reincarnation. King Asoka (250 B.C.) made great efforts to protect the sacred cow. He set up veterinary hospitals and staffed them with state-paid salihatrya. Horses, elephants, birds, and fish, as well as cattle, received medical attention. Today, India is the only country that has sanctuaries for old and decrepit animals. The laws not only protect the animals, but they impose the death penalty on anyone who kills a cow or an elephant.

During these thousands of years, the world has passed through many medical fads. The demon theory of disease was the first recognized speculation on the cause of illness in both men and animals, and this same reasoning still holds in many areas of the world today. In some civilizations, demons were driven off into the fog and darkness by the beating of drums. In others, animals, and to a lesser extent human beings, were sacrificed to appease the evil spirits. The casting of spells and the use of charms as health cures are sometimes heeded even today. With such a background, it is not surprising that signs, charms, mixtures of dung, urine, and evil-smelling extracts were the principal ingredients prescribed in ancient times.

Like simple attempts at healing, primitive surgery was useless and risky. One of the first operations consisted of trephining, or cutting a hole in the skull with a stone knife to permit the escape of evil spirits.

In the history of the Hebrews, we find that they considered disease to be a punishment for sin. Moses set forth rules of sanitation and segregated the sick, but he discouraged treatment. Medicine did not advance very rapidly under his code and the people had little need for doctors either for their animals or for themselves. Later, when the Jews came under the influence of the political supremacy of Greece, the priests became health officers and the status of physicians improved. The Hebrews were good shepherds and herdsmen, and their wealth was measured by the number of animals they owned.

Persia also considered medicine to be in the realm of the priest-physician. Disease was still thought to be due to evil spirits, and special rites were required for the purification of any who had contacted the dead or infected. Bodies were usually left to be consumed by vultures rather than buried.

In Greece, Hippocrates (460 B.C. to 377 B.C.) used few of the mysterious and revolting prescriptions of the Egyptians and others. His methods were simple and natural, following the philosophy, "Do no harm if you cannot do good." He emphasized nutritious diet, suitable climate, exercise, and good hygiene. Such practice is the mark of a good physician and veterinarian today. However, Hippocrates and his contemporaries did no postmortems on humans: hence there was little known about anatomy and physiology. What little information there was came from studying animals, which created many misconceptions as far as human beings were concerned.

After Hippocrates came Aristotle (382 B.C. to 322 B.C.), who dissected many species and recorded anatomical information about most domestic animals. He also studied embryonated eggs, developed theories about circulation, designated the body regions, and named the parts of the body. It was he who discovered that the horse had no gall bladder. His chart on determining the age of horses by their teeth is very accurate. Aristotle mentions such diseases as tetanus, intense breathing (heaves), abscesses of the throat (strangles), barley disease (laminitis), and gives an account of how castration should be performed.

Roman and Byzantine Periods (200 B.C. to 500 A.D.)

For several centuries, until the Greek influence was felt, medicine received little attention as such in Rome, and illness was favored with attention only by superstitious magicians and midwives. The Greek writings were heeded then to some extent, but there is nothing in the records to show that veterinary medicine advanced.

Following the fall of the Roman Empire when the capital was moved to Constantinople (Byzantium), the period known as the Byzantine Age was an era of major progress for veterinary medicine. Apsyrtus was a chief contributor to the "Hippiatrika," a collection of veterinary writings. This was the first good work on such things as the digestive troubles of horses, surgical procedures in which ligation and cautery were employed, splinting fractures, and recognizing and treating tetanus. "Hippiatrika" was translated into Latin, and it is known that the Roman Vegetius borrowed from it heavily when he wrote his "Books of the Veterinary Art."

Thus, credit is due to Apsyrtus and others, but Vegetius is often referred to as the "Father of Veterinary Medicine." Although his work was not original, he rewrote much that was worthy of preservation and added many personal and valuable observations. He was the first to recommend fumigation of stables to control contagion, and he had the courage to contend that disease was not always a sign of divine displeasure but often could be attributed to negligence of the animal owner.

Unfortunately, these writings were all lost to civilization during the Dark Ages and it was not until 1572 that the first translation of Vegetius' work appeared.

The Middle Ages (500 A.D. to 1500 A.D.)

In the Middle Ages, men became slaves to convention guided largely by the prevailing philosophy of the Church. Men were denied the right to heal and medicine returned to the status of the temple healing of ancient Greece. All dissection and surgery—that is, most experimentation and thus progress—were forbidden, and the better minds of the time turned to law and other such professions. The Church by her incantations and superstitions, exercised a grip over animal medicine which discouraged research. This dark curtain was slow in lifting. Paradoxically, it should be noted, throughout this period monks preserved medical literature. They also were the first to apply the concept of hospitals established to care for the sick. Many of these had clean, airy accommodations, a good water supply, and sanitation systems.

The Renaissance (1500 A.D. to 1700 A.D.)

The Renaissance brought creativity, vigorous activity, freedom of thought, a better philosophy for living, and a receptive attitude toward innovation. The invention of printing was probably one important key to this. Private schools were established to teach the art of treating animals, and in most of the countries a system of licensure to practice was set up in recognition of those who became proficient in these skills. This was a golden age for discoveries and new ideas.

When Harvey, in 1628, discovered the vascular circulation, he pointed up the need to look closely at the tissues of the body. Then Leuwenhoek, making his own lens, put together a microscope that enabled him to see red blood cells and later to describe bacteria.

The Eighteenth and Nineteenth Centuries

Lancisi, the physician to the Pope in 1715, rid Rome of rinderpest* by setting up strict measures of animal control. Movements of animals from infected districts was prohibited under penalty of death. Dead animals were taken and buried in quicklime without being skinned. No one was allowed to treat sick animals. Only meat inspected and stamped with a hot iron could be sold. No cattle or dogs were allowed to enter areas where there were sick animals. Healthy cattle were removed from pastures where sick animals had been grazing, and these pastures were quarantined and regarded as contaminated. The feed and water vessels were cleaned with quicklime and the clothes of the shepherds were fumigated. All trade in cattle was arrested during the outbreak. In nine months, these strict measures were responsible for eliminating the disease.

At this time, all of Europe was in need of control laws, for it was estimated that in four years 1,500,000 head of cattle were lost because of cattle plague in western Europe alone. The rest of Europe took little heed of the value gained from isolation in Rome and over 200,000,000 head of cattle died between 1711 and 1769 because of lack of traffic control in cattle marketing.

In 1714, the plague crossed the channel into England. A cure by medicine was sought, but no provision was made

---
* A virus disease of cattle.

for isolation. This allowed the virus to spread over England before the public became aroused enough to adopt laws to control the movement of cattle. Opinion was divided on what should be done, but finally the government got around to passing strict laws over slaughter and control. This stopped the epidemic, but the losses were extreme for the cattle owners. The government, realizing the great hardship this brought to the farmers, provided indemnity for those suffering a loss. This may not have been the first time a government paid animal owners indemnity for their losses, but it was the largest allowance any government had ever declared. This experience was a costly one for farmers and government alike, and it paved the way for quick and strict government action in all future outbreaks.

Canine distemper* became known as a distinct disease about 1750 when two types, respiratory and epileptic forms, were recognized. This disease reappeared and destroyed whole kennels year after year when pups were four, five, and six months of age. There is no record of any control for this until years later.

Pleuropneumonia, glanders, rinderpest, anthrax, and many other infections continued to make an appearance almost out of nowhere. The cause of each one was not known, and the obstinate adherence to the humoral theory of pathology delayed improvement in ridding the herds and flocks of these infections. The humoral theory was that the body contained four humors—blood, phlegm, yellow bile, and black bile, and that when these were mixed in the right proportions an animal or a human had good health; im-

---

* Canine Distemper, a virus disease of dogs. Pleuropneumonia, a contagious pneumonia of cattle affecting the pleura as the lungs. Glanders, a contagious bacterial disease of horses. Anthrax, a dark carbuncle that resembled a piece of coal caused by anthrax bacteria that affects all mammals.

proper proportions or irregular distribution constituted disease. Blood-letting, which was an attempt to balance the humors, was a universal therapeutic method in both human and animal medicine well into the twentieth century. The formula of isolation and slaughter to eliminate an infectious disease was well known, but politicians and rich animal owners opposed such measures unless an outbreak became severe enough to threaten the entire animal population. Individual cases were treated with ancient prescriptions, remedies, and superstitions that had been futilely practiced for 2,000 years.

The first real headway toward controlling disease by vaccination occurred in England. In 1796, Edward Jenner, a physician, took particular note of a common observation among rural folk: that dairymaids who had had cowpox would not contract smallpox. He began an extensive inquiry into cowpox, but it was twenty years before he brought to fruition his idea of vaccination. He was honored throughout the world, and still is, for this wonderful piece of work. Jenner contributed much to veterinary medicine both in his inquiries into animal diseases and by the nature of his writings, which set forth his methods of analysis.

In the mid-eighteenth century in France, a need for veterinary education was recognized. It was decided that the irregular manner of handling disease for the previous forty years had been fruitless, and that it was about time to give the diseases of animals a scientific approach. Accordingly, a school of veterinary medicine was established in 1761 in Lyons, and in 1766 a second school was set up at Alfort. In 1825, a third school opened at Toulouse, and here primary attention was given to cattle and sheep in contrast to the earlier schools where the cases were mainly horses.

The Veterinary College of London was established in 1791. Unfortunately, the philosophy of some of the men who directed it for many years favored limiting education so that veterinarians could not achieve the prestige accorded physicians. Graduates were little more than practically trained stable hands and horse-shoers. This situation did not improve until Youatt became active in the 1830s, and the Veterinary College of London began to earn the prestige that it has as an educational institution today.

Earlier Edinburgh was fortunate in having William Dick, a man of unusual ability. He founded the Edinburgh Veterinary College and even the first set of buildings was built with his money in 1833. He selected and trained men of high caliber, seven of whom became deans of veterinary schools in the United Kingdom and America. It was one of his students, Monro, an anatomist in the medical school at Edinburgh, who devised a stomach tube of flexible iron wire covered with leather for cattle bloat in 1779. The tube was shoved down the throat of a bloated cow and the gas was allowed to escape through the tube.

In 1814, Peall of Ireland recognized a difference between the flu-like diseases of glanders and strangles (abscesses of the throat) in the horse. This difference was verified scientifically by the introduction of the Mallein test in 1890.

Early in the nineteenth century, veterinarians began to come to America from foreign colleges, mostly in England. A veterinary college was established in Philadelphia in 1852. In Canada the Ontario Veterinary College was established in 1862. Before the turn of the century, twenty-five veterinary colleges, most of them private institutions, were launched in America. The first state school was established at Iowa State University in 1879. Gradually the private schools disappeared and were replaced by state schools, which were larger and much better supported through agricultural interests.

In the last half of the nineteenth century, the horse still remained king as far as veterinary practice was concerned. The introduction of steam railways caused many veterinarians to give thought to the future of the profession and some even feared the bicycle would put them out of work. It almost seemed disloyal for a veterinarian to learn to drive an automobile in the early 1900s. Despite these fears and rumors, there has been a steadily increasing demand for the veterinarian through the years.

Had it not been for outbreaks of foot-and-mouth* disease, pleuropneumonia, and sheep pox,** the study of cattle and sheep pathology might have been delayed even longer. A series of these devastating outbreaks caused the American public to cry for more and better qualified veterinarians. Vigorous measures were finally taken to control the importation and the distribution of animals. Increased knowledge and better methods were continually introduced. Even so, therapeutics in both man and animals suffered from such absurdities as bloodletting. Rivers of blood were drawn by opening a large vein, usually the jugular, with elaborate instruments designed to cut the vessel. Animals were bled until they stumbled. In spite of their weakened condition, many of them recovered, although not because of the surgery.

The first animal disease outbreak to engage the attention of the American public was Texas fever. This was introduced by cattle from the Spanish colonies of Mexico which had been imported from the West Indies around 1610. By

---
* Foot and mouth disease, a virus disease of clove-footed animals.
** Sheep pox, a virus disease causing an eruptive lesion on the skin.

1790, cattle coming from south of the border had filtered into native herds in the Southern states and as far north as North Carolina. The losses from Texas fever were so great that in 1795 North Carolina passed the first state law restricting the movement of livestock. Pennsylvania and Maryland also had heavy losses as a result of this infection.

For many years, Texas fever baffled scientific minds. Healthy cattle quickly died after they came in contact with local cattle from infected areas. It was soon recognized that losses from this illness were seasonal and always occurred between the months of April and November. Several states passed laws prohibiting the movement of cattle across state lines during these months. In 1893, Smith, Kilborne, and Custice discovered the cause of Texas fever to be in a small parasite that invaded the red blood cells. It was also discovered that this parasite was carried by the cattle tick. The cattle tick hibernated in cold weather, which accounted for the seasonal occurrence of the disease. Once this was understood, quarantine stations and disinfection and dipping stations got rid of the ticks. In a relatively short time, cattle ceased dying and the disease was brought under control.

This discovery of insects as disease carriers not only saved the cattle, but it gave new life to research, which ultimately brought control of malaria, yellow fever, typhus, bubonic plague, and many other diseases which are carried by insects.

In 1833, hog cholera first appeared in Ohio, and for three-quarters of a century this disease ravaged the hog industry because there was no medicine to prevent it. By the early 1900s, cholera spread through the corn belt and entire herds of hogs died in the epidemic that followed. I can remember as a youngster seeing big fires burning at night on many of the adjoining farms to consume the carcasses of hogs that had died during the day. A ray of hope came when a promising serum was developed that gave immunity for short periods of time. By 1920, the effective use of the vaccine was well enough established to insure pork for the American table. This vaccine, and its successors, have been so effective that now the disease has entirely been eliminated from the United States. Without an effective vaccine and the use of special quarantine measures ham and bacon would be very scarce on our tables today.

The next infectious disease to arouse national concern —a contagion called pleuropneumonia*—afflicted the cattle in this country in 1843. A lone cow with this disease was imported from Germany, unloaded from the ship in New York harbor, and taken to a stable in Brooklyn. From this single cow pleuropneumonia spread very quickly and most of the cattle on Long Island were wiped out. It took four years to control this costly outbreak. There was no cure or prevention for the disease, for vaccines had not yet been discovered. After several meetings of high-ranking officials, it was decided that in order to protect the uninfected valuable cattle in the United States, all the infected and exposed animals must be sacrificed and their carcasses destroyed by burial under the ground in quicklime. Such a decision was not popular to the owners who were forced to destroy their animals. However, the disease did disappear, and this method for controlling a potentially disastrous disease is still the method of choice when an infection strikes. For example, three times foot-and-mouth disease has threatened the cattle population of this country since 1870, and each time keen observation and hard work by the veterinarians,

---

* A contagious disease of cattle.

using the same quarantine and slaughter method which was effective against pleuropneumonia, have made it possible to eliminate this dread virus disease.

The Twentieth Century

With the settling of America and the establishment of the livestock industry came the task of transporting food animals to market. At first, they were brought to market on foot, but with the establishment of cross-country railroad-stock cars were built to transport animals to the central markets. The methods of livestock shipping were crude and hazardous, as could be expected, and losses from shipping were alarming. However, the time saved and the ease of effort seemed to overbalance the loss by death and loss from decrease of flesh. But as the number and value of livestock increased, the annual loss was felt more and more. In 1919, after seventy years of shipping by rail, the annual loss was estimated to be $5,000,000.

At this time, veterinarians played an important role in the establishment of a Livestock Loss Prevention Board. Losses and abuses in shipping were so bad that one hog in 300, one bovine animal in 1,100, and one sheep in 850 were dead upon delivery. Losses were reduced by the passage of the 28-hour law, which meant that all animals had to be unloaded, watered, fed, and rested after being loaded in a car for over 28 hours. This, coupled with improved bedding in cars to prevent injury from quick stops and a jerky ride, lowered the losses until by 1933 they were reduced by one-half or better.

Even many years earlier it was obvious to concerned legislators that some policing agency backed up by strong law was necessary to protect the animals of the United

States. We have celebrated the centennial of the 1865 law dealing with the importation and interstate shipment of animals. After one hundred years, it is more important than ever. Modern world transportation by air, rail, highway, and water constantly shuffles the livestock to far-distant points, and with each move there is constant danger of admitting and spreading a disease new to the area of consignment.

Veterinarians responsible for administering control of the movement of livestock are called regulatory veterinarians. Approximately 4,000 work in this capacity for federal, state, and local governments, and they are responsible for controlling the spread of over one hundred diseases that affect man as well as livestock. There are 1,200 regulatory veterinarians engaged in food inspection; the remainder are in the military service or other specialized branches of regulatory service, which include control of the production and marketing of serums, vaccines, drugs, and other biological products for animal use.

In 1890, a system of federal meat inspection was established making it a law that only meat that has had inspection under the supervision of federal veterinarians could be sold for interstate shipment. This law has provided us with the safest and most edible meat supply in the world.

Veterinarians have a notable record for assisting in the control and irradication of diseases transmitted from animal to man. In 1917, a bovine tuberculosis program was launched. Research revealed that the disease in cattle was spread to man through milk and meat. At that time, tuberculosis sanitariums were crowded with patients, and others sick with the disease were waiting admittance. The hunchback, who used to be a familiar figure on the street, is now seldom seen. This deformity occurred as a result of tuberculosis of the spine. The elimination of tuberculosis in cattle, plus the discovery of effective drugs to treat the disease, have decreased the incidence to the point where today many of our tuberculosis sanitariums are no longer needed.

Veterinarians played a major role in this battle for good health. In the 1920s, between 50,000 and 70,000 cattle and hogs were condemned with tuberculosis and considered unfit for food. Since that time, there have been conscientious programs for testing and eliminating infected animals. Today, as a result of this program, less than 250 cattle with this disease are condemned each year. This means that bovine tuberculosis has been practically eliminated in America. Veterinarians have not only stopped the spread of tuberculosis among cattle, hogs, and poultry, but they have helped to eliminate this dread disease in man.

Undulant fever, also known as Bang's disease or brucellosis, causes abortion in cattle, goats, and hogs, and a chronic flu-like illness in man. The disease is transmitted from animal to animal by direct contact and to man by contact with the affected animal or through the milk. In 1933, a coöperative campaign was started to control the spread of the disease and to eventually eliminate it altogether. Today a majority of the states, Puerto Rico, and the Virgin Islands have modified, certified brucellosis-free areas. In addition, 56 counties in individual states and the whole state of New Hampshire are brucellosis-free. Brucellosis in cattle is controlled by calfhood vaccination and restricted interchange of breeding animals. More than six million calves are vaccinated annually, and all breeding cattle must be blood-tested when sold.

Loss of animals from disease and death directly attributable to parasites is estimated to cause animal losses of over a billion dollars. No estimate can be made of the loss in feed that was wasted on these animals or of the loss in pounds of flesh caused to animals that survived. The parasite problem, while partially controlled, is still a challenge.

In one instance, however, a serious problem that has resulted in saving thousands of animals has been solved. For many years, the screw-worm fly caused death and crippling damage to animals in the Southeast. The damage started when the screw-worm fly laid its eggs on open wounds of living animals. Larvae then hatched from these eggs and burrowed into the muscle beneath the wounds. Toxins from the larvae themselves caused the flesh to slough away and, if the wound was not cared for, the animal died. In an effort to control the flies, it was found that atomic radiation could be used to make the worms sterile. A screw-worm fly mates only once, the male then dies, and the female dies when the eggs are laid. If the eggs fail to hatch in a given area, the over-all fly population is thus depleted. The regular release of a million sterile flies, which mingled and mated with the native fertile screw-worm flies, brought a successful reduction in the screw-worm population, and it may be that they will disappear altogether.

Since the time of Pasteur, veterinary science has been marked by a succession of discoveries that have had the effect of greatly reducing the hazards of animal life and production. Specific viruses and bacteria and parasites have been found to be the causes. More recently, nutritional disturbances, poisoning from plants, and toxic drugs have been pinpointed as the causes of still other groups of diseases.

As an example, the conquest in 1913 of blackleg, a disease that annually took a heavy toll of cattle, was a dramatic step forward in the progress of veterinary medicine. In river valley pastures each spring as cattle were taken out to graze, many of the animals, particularly the young ones, would become lame. In a few hours the limb would swell to about twice its normal size and the animal would die in a very short time. When the skin was removed from the leg, the flesh was found to be full of air bubbles and a sweet aroma, somewhat like rancid butter, would come from the affected parts. The muscle that was affected would be dark brown or black in color—hence the name of the disease.

On making a cross-section of the muscle, it was found that there were many small air spaces. Under a microscope it was discovered that a bacteria was present that belonged to the family of spore formers. This meant that the spores had a protective coat that would preserve them for years. probably even for centuries, and the organisms would remain alive in the soil. This disease is only encountered in the lowlands, as in the Missouri River bottom land where it was a serious problem for many years. Each year after heavy spring rains, some of these organisms are washed up and any cattle that are not immune will succumb to the disease if they become infected.

The first vaccine against blackleg was produced by impregnating a string or thread with a few organisms. The string was drawn through the animal's skin with a needle, causing a slight infection. This set up a slow reaction that built up antibodies against the disease and rendered the animal immune to further attacks. Later, a vaccine was developed in the form of a tiny pellet into which a few spores were placed. This pellet was injected under the skin of cattle and they developed a light case of the disease. Within a few more years the organisms could be grown on artificial media; these were killed and a liquid vaccine was produced that could be administered with a syringe. This method is still in use. Thus were the teachings of Jenner, Pasteur, and other pioneers turned to good account in conquering this and many other animal diseases.

In view of the many spectacular conquests of diseases since the beginning of history to the present time, it would seem that we would have all the answers, but this is not true. The threat of disease is continuous and there are now a host of new diseases such as radiation sickness and staphylococcus infections, which are an inadvertent consequence of man's scientific advances. In the nation's capital and elsewhere the best-trained men in biological sciences are spending long hours trying to solve these new problems in animal disease control.

Three different virus diseases claim attention and concentrated effort in veterinary research at present. All three have existed throughout the years in small, isolated areas and a little knowledge, money, and effort could have eliminated all three. But, because of national barriers, jealousies, and reluctance on the part of some countries to help less fortunate neighbors, these diseases have now spread and have become a threat to the world's livestock.

Rinderpest, mentioned several times in this chapter, is still such a threat to the international cattle population that it is inadvisable to import cattle to this country for fear that they may be carriers.

African swine fever, for decades confined to a few sparsely populated African communities, now threatens the swine population of Europe and Asia. Unfortunately, modern air transportation may have been the means of scattering the virus.

Some of the horses of Africa harbor a virus which produces a respiratory and circulatory illness, usually fatal, known as African horse sickness. At one time, this affected only a few horses in one small country of Africa. When it was recognized, a small amount of work and the money to pay indemnity for the disposal of a relatively few animals would probably have eliminated this disease from the world. But this challenge was not met and since World War II horses from this area have been shipped to Asia, the Middle East, and the Far East, causing this virus to spread and resulting in tremendous losses of animals.

A few years ago the United States had to weigh the diplomatic problem of whether to permit the acceptance of a horse given by a ruler in Pakistan as a gift to the wife of our President. The danger that this horse may be a carrier of the dreaded African horse sickness, to which our horses have no immunity, is a very grave one. A quarantine imposed for the safety of our animals solved that problem.

Currently, cattlemen want to import new breeds of cattle from Europe. Most European countries still have active cases of foot and mouth disease. Importing live cattle or even semen to breed our native cattle imposes great dangers to our bovine population because animals that carry no immunity to this disease are especially suseptible. An outbreak of this disease could cost millions of dollars.

So as man continues to migrate around the world and into outer space, he creates new disease climates that affect him and all the other creatures of the earth. This is the challenge offered to the young scientists in all fields of medicine today. There is no doubt that these problems will be as difficult, as heartbreaking, and eventually as rewarding to solve as any of those reported on these pages.

CHAPTER II

The Diseases of Animals

In the course of becoming acquainted with veterinary medicine, people are often surprised to find that there is so much illness among animals, and the interested inquirer often asks such questions as, "What diseases do animals have?" "Are they the same diseases as seen in man?" "Do animals have cancer?" In answering these questions, let us recall that all mammals, regardless of size, have a comparable skeleton and a set of organs which have the same functions and similar cells as those of man. Thus, it stands to reason that the diseases of lower animals and man are similar.

Some illnesses originate within the body. These are either metabolic, endocrine, degenerative, or neoplastic in nature. Metabolic diseases are those resulting from faulty physical and chemical processes of the organs. For example, if the pancreas does not function properly, not enough sugar is converted into usable form; as a result, the patient, whether animal or man, suffers from diabetes. Or, if the kidney function fails, toxic waste products build up in the blood and the patient, animal or man, has nephritis, or Bright's disease (kidney disease).

The endocrine glands have as their function the production of hormones. These are catalytic body regulators and if these are not produced in proper amounts, the result may be dwarfism, giantism, goiter, or a reproductive failure.

Organ degeneration is associated with old age and each animal has its own pattern for this. Each species varies in size, shape, and life purpose, and its metabolic rate is geared accordingly. The smaller the animals, the more rapid is the metabolic rate and, with some exceptions, the shorter the life span. For example, the mouse is very small, his heart beats very rapidly, his metabolism is very high, and his life span can be measured in months. The metabolic rate of the dog is lower and the life span is longer, about thirteen years on an average. The dog matures rapidly though, and by the end of the first year is sexually mature and can produce young. By the tenth or eleventh year the dog's hair is turning gray and by the thirteenth year he is senile. Among larger animals the horse, for instance, reaches about twenty-four years of age before death overtakes him. Man's life span is still measured by the traditional three score and ten years.

Then, in addition to metabolic, endocrine, and degenerative changes, all animals are subject to neoplastic or tumorus diseases. Cancer in man and all animals is very similar, and scientists have benefited greatly from a better understanding of tumors by having an opportunity to study this disease in lower animals. The mouse, whose life span is very short, is used to study cancer through several generations of a given family in a matter of a few years. A considerable amount of knowledge about cancer has been obtained in this way.

Diseases caused by external living agents such as bacteria, protozoa, fungi, and viruses are responsible for most of the infectious diseases; hog cholera and blackleg are examples.

Organisms not only attack the body and cause disturbances of function to the individual animal, but they may be transmitted and cause disease in other animals. Luckily for the continuation of our existence and that of other animals, most diseases affect only one species. This specificity makes it easier to control disease outbreaks. However, a few diseases such as rabies, anthrax, brucellosis and tuberculosis attack all animals.

Disease is spread in many ways. Some of them have unique cycles, but most are spread by: (1) direct contact between susceptible and diseased animals; (2) contact through fomites, which are inanimate contaminated objects such as implements, trucks, feed sacks, litter, or the clothing of the caretakers; (3) contact with a disease carrier such as an animal that has developed a tolerance to an infection so that it remains well but carries the disease organisms and spreads them to susceptible animals; (4) infection from contaminated soil in which the bacteria spores and fungi may have lived for an indefinite period and then produce a disease when contacted by susceptible animals (tetanus, anthrax, and histoplasmosis); (5) contaminated food and water; (6) airborne organisms inhaled by animals; (7) bloodsucking parasites that live on animals, thus absorbing living agents from a sick animal's blood and transmitting them to other animals (heart worms and anaplasmosis are transmitted in this fashion); and (8) bacteria found in normal surroundings which will produce disease if the animal's resistance is lowered or if the protective skin is broken (staphylococcal wound infections are an example).

Besides all the infections that may be acquired, there are hazardous environmental circumstances such as injury, stress, extreme heat and burns, cold, chemical poisons, and nutritional deficiencies that cause illnesses. Treating injuries comprises a large part of the services rendered in any veterinary practice. Fractures and wounds are very frequent in all classes of animals. In this motorized age, for example, dogs allowed to run unleashed are often the victims of accidents due to tractors, motorcycles, and automobiles.

Environmental changes have produced a whole new group of diseases. The cow by nature produces enough milk to feed her calf, but since milk products are a good source of food for man, the cow has been bred to increase her milk production so that she not only has enough food for her calf but also supplies milk, butter, and cheese for man. It is not surprising that mastitis, a stress disease affecting the udder, is a major problem in dairy herds.

Similarly, the hen has been converted into a bird that not only produces enough eggs to raise a nest of chickens, but to supply the breakfast table of the nation as well. In addition, the broiler is forced to develop rapidly to supply meat for the table. These added stresses bring many health problems that need the attention of the veterinarian.

Then there are the toxic effects of many new chemical products used today to treat the soil and to control insects, bacteria, and fungi. Many of these chemicals are toxic not only to the insects and weeds they are designed to kill, but also to man and animals. With every new chemical marketed, a new disease problem may arise.

When increased production in either plant or animal is demanded, vitamins, minerals, proteins, and carbohydrates are needed in large quantities. Failure to maintain a proper balance of these products causes associated nutritional diseases such as rickets and scurvy. Whenever production is increased, the veterinarian must be at hand to see that there is a balance maintained or disease is the result.

These, then, are the diseases from which animals suffer;

some are natural, but many are man-made. Disease control and animal husbandry offer an ever-increasing challenge to the veterinarian in modern practice. The greater the demand for production, the greater the challenge for the veterinarian to see that the nation and the world are fed and that the animals receive a maximum of protection in the process.

There are many warnings that the world is on the brink of a famine so large and inexorable that more people will die than have been killed in all wars in history.

Veterinarians will be given the challenge of helping increase the animal protein supply to reduce the catastrophe. It is clear that the United States must play a vital role in alleviating the effects of world famine.

CHAPTER III

Qualifications

After this introduction to the history and the scope of the profession, you will probably ask yourself, "Am I suited to this kind of a career?" Perhaps I can make formulating an opinion easier by telling you of some of the qualifications I have observed in young men and women who have become excellent veterinarians, and by encouraging you to become personally acquainted with members of the profession so you can judge these facts for yourself.

Veterinarians have an intense concern and affection for animals. In addition, even as youngsters they had a respect for and a dedication to animal life that reached far beyond the average. For example, during my years of large-animal practice, it was common in the hot summer to vaccinate pigs for hog cholera in the early morning when it was still cool, so the pigs would not become overheated from handling. This meant leaving the office for the country about five o'clock in the morning. A likeable young boy, Jim by name, became so interested in going to the country with me that every morning at this early hour he would be at my office waiting to help load the car and go along to vaccinate the pigs. At other times, he would forsake his pals and a ball game for a trip to the country to treat an animal. His interest was genuine, his love for animals real. He went on through college to become a veterinarian who is now a credit to his profession and his community.

Another good veterinarian, Dr. Frank by name, was a farm boy who gathered in every orphaned or injured pig and lamb he could find. He would often get up at night to see that these animals were fed, dry, and warm. As I write this, there is a young lad in our neighborhood who is devoted to wild life. He has a turtle sanctuary and an aquarium where he harbors frogs eggs until they hatch. He goes to great lengths to learn about the habits of these animals. Though only ten years old, he is a good candidate for veterinary medicine.

During my years in small-animal practice, I regularly employed high school boys and girls to work in our hospital after school and on Saturdays. The students applying for these jobs always professed a love for animals, but it was those who actually owned one or two pets and wanted to assume the responsibility of feeding and exercising them who had the greatest devotion to their jobs.

I recall that once we had a litter of newly born puppies left without a mother to care for them. Three of our high school girl employees asked if they could raise these puppies. It was in the summer and the three were working full time, but they volunteered to take turns caring for these pups at home at night. This meant setting an alarm and getting up every three hours to feed them individually with a nursing bottle. Each girl maintained her vigil with enthusiasm until the pups were old enough to be able to go all night without feeding. These youngsters have the sincere love of animals and respect for life that it takes to succeed in a career in veterinary medicine.

The ability to adapt and discipline oneself to the degree that the welfare of animals has a very high priority is one of the primary requisites for success in this profession. It is this desire to serve others that is so important. You must ask yourself, "Am I sincerely interested in devoting my life to animals, or am I just temporarily attracted to some aspect of the profession?"

What about your family? Will they be sympathetic toward your leading a life of service to animals? Will they give you encouragement? This understanding is important because it is a long, hard grind to complete, first, the pre-veterinary college years and, then, the four more years of professional training. Since college is an expensive undertaking, it is important that the family's attitude be one of sympathy and ungrudging financial support. Then, when you as a veterinarian have a family of your own, your wife and children must be sympathetic and understanding. There will be some missed trips, birthday parties, evenings out, and picnics, which the family must endure. If the family will not tolerate this service-above-self philosophy, the career may not progress as well as it should. Service is responsibility, and the true professional man has the desire and devotion to endure disappointments and to love his work despite its obstacles.

One must be a good enough student to qualify for and absorb a medical education. If you frequently want to know "why" and are the kind who seeks more information and likes to solve problems, then veterinary medicine will offer you a chance to develop and satisfy this kind of intellectual curiosity.

The individual seeking this career must also think in terms of health and physical endurance. Do you enjoy hard physical work and long hours? Can you work hard for several days with only a few hours of sleep? Are you subject to illnesses that keep you from the job? Your sick patients will come first and must be attended daily.

In summary, some people would consider the long and irregular hours a very undesirable feature, but those of us who love our work and the profession feel that these are really not sacrifices and inconveniences at all. Most doctors have enough interest and curiosity that they would rather be diagnosing an ailment and treating a sick animal than trying to make a grand slam at a bridge table.

One of the best ways to learn more about the profession is to become acquainted with several veterinarians. Start by getting acquainted with one or more in your vicinity. A veterinarian is usually very willing and eager to help prospective veterinary students. His advice is valuable because sometime in the last twenty years he successfully combated and surmounted all of the problems that are now facing you, and the story of how he accomplished this may hold some of the keys to the solution of your problems. He will tell you about his school. He will be acquainted with many veterinarians from other schools and from the exchange of knowledge with his colleagues he will know the advantages of different veterinary schools. He will also spend time discussing pre-veterinary training.

Become acquainted with more than one veterinarian. No two are alike; each one has a different personality, a different philosophy, and a different plan for the future. In making acquaintance with a veterinarian, you will be more successful if your introduction and approach are well planned. The following are some suggestions:

A. Find names of veterinarians.

1. Arrange for an introduction through a mutual friend.
2. Consult the yellow pages of the telephone book.
3. Phone and request an appointment to discuss the veterinary profession. Find out when the veterinarian can see you.
4. Be sure that you are well groomed when you keep your appointment. Wear business attire. Remember that the veterinarian will discourage you if your appearance is not that of a good professional prospect.
5. Plan your interview carefully. Take along a pen and pad to write down needed information.
6. Be on time or early; don't keep the veterinarian waiting.

B. Proposed questions to ask the veterinarian during the interview.
   1. What is veterinary medicine?
   2. What is the future of the profession?
   3. Would he take veterinary medinice if he were to start over again?
   4. What about the success of this business?
   5. From what college did he graduate? Year?
   6. What is the best way to be admitted to a veterinary college?
   7. What subjects should you take in high school?
   8. At what school should the pre-veterinary years be taken?
   9. What veterinary colleges would he recommend?
   10. Does he know the dean or any faculty members you might contact if you should visit the school he recommends?

11. What does he estimate it costs per year to go to a veterinary school?
12. What is school like? Have him describe the scope of the training offered.
13. Ask him if you might return to watch him do his work at some appointed time.
14. Be sure to thank him for his time and courtesies to you.

Another good way to become acquainted with the activities of veterinary medicine is to assist a veterinarian with his work. There are many odd jobs a high school student would enjoy that would be helpful to the doctor. A part-time job at a veterinary hospital or with a large-animal practitioner will afford you an opportunity to find out how you like the work. If, by chance, the veterinarian does not have work for you, ask him whether, on your own, you may spend some time in his office. If he lets you come in, do not make a nuisance of yourself, but try to do helpful chores that might repay him for the time he has given you.

In large-animal practice an assistant can bring the gear and instruments to and from the car. The equipment will have to be cleaned and returned while the veterinarian discusses the case with the client. During the procedure of treating animals at the farm, the assistant can fill syringes, write down data for case histories, and hold instruments during operations. Back at the office, an assistant can make himself useful while getting ready for the next call by replacing soiled instruments, replenishing drugs and vaccines in the emergency bag, laying out a new set of sterile instruments and syringes, and getting a change of clothing ready for the doctor.

In a small-animal hospital, teenagers, both boys and

girls, are often needed to exercise and feed the animals and as substitutes on evenings, Saturdays, and holidays when the regular receptionist is off duty. Since getting a college education is expensive, such jobs are not only beneficial as experience, but the money earned will help the student meet the costs of his education.

CHAPTER IV

Veterinary Education

The degree of D.V.M. or V.M.D., doctor of veterinary medicine, takes a minimum of 7 years of college work. This is also true of other medical sciences, such as dentistry. To get an M.D., one must take an even longer course of study. From this book, and from what your high school counselors and others may have said, you undoubtedly have decided that getting into a professional school is not an easy task. This is true, but do not be discouraged. Twenty-five hundred students are accepted into the veterinary colleges each year. Why not you? The secret of being admitted is to follow a well-planned program for reaching this goal. Prepare your strategy now.

Getting through school will be hard work and you can expect some stumbling blocks to slow down your progress. In the normal course of the 7 or 8 years, it would be rare indeed if one did not encounter some personal or family illness, some financial reverses, or some difficulty in meeting all the scholastic requirements. But if you have a definite goal in mind, you will be better equipped to overcome any setbacks or disappointments. By now, you know your strong and weak points academically, and financially so take pains to plan accordingly.

Choosing a School

An applicant for admission to a veterinary school has very little choice in the school he will attend. The demand for admission is so great and the cost of training so costly, that the schools themselves have had to limit their students to the state where the veterinary school is located and to states where special arrangements have been made for accepting students.

There is good reason for this, since a student's tuition pays only a fraction of the cost of his education, and the school must rely heavily on funds from state taxes to pay its budget. This obligates the school to take most of its students from the state furnishing the funds, and if out of state students are taken, supplemental funds must be paid for the students' cost of training. Most schools see the need to share their teaching facilities with joining states, and therefore contractural arrangements are made between the school and the participating state to train a limited number of their students.

States having a contract with a veterinary school agree to pay a specific sum per year per student for the student's training. Veterinary education costs from three to eight times more than the cost of the regular tuition, and under the contract the state sending students pay most of the difference between what the students pay in tuition and the cost of their education.

To be sure, there are disadvantages to limiting admissions to specific areas. Even though the curricula are similar, schools in certain areas excel in special disciplines. This is usually due to the demands for certain services and the emphasis placed upon specific diseases or conditions in a region. For example, Texas A. & M. University ranks high in range cattle diseases, Iowa State University excels in swine problems, Cornell University offers an unusual amount of training in dairy cattle problems, and here at the University of Pennsylvania is located the world's largest and most advanced horse clinic.

These facts need not worry the student seeking admission to a veterinary school because the training is excellent in all schools. Schools, on an exchange basis, will send interested students during their final year or during resident training to schools offering more training in a specific field.

Students anticipating making an application to a veterinary school should get specific information about where and how they can be admitted to the school available to them. The Department of Education of their specific state should be able to supply this information. The veterinary school available for residents of a state should be contacted for a school catalogue and for information about making an application.

When the students have studied these, it is well to discuss the process of making an application with as many knowledgeable people as possible. Again for this, the local veterinarians should have many helpful ideas on this. Those students who make excellent grades, that have worthwhile plans for developing experiences and data that show desire and motivation toward veterinary medicine are the ones that always attract the eye of the Admissions Committee. The students who work and plan in this manner will be rewarded when an application is made.

It is recommended that the prospective applicants not limit their scope of interest to any specific area of veterinary medicine. It is too early in experiences to be definite to the point of closing ones' mind to other fields. As students horizons broaden with experience and education, many preconceived ideas change.

Qualifications for Admission

For the moment, pretend that you are the chairman of the Admissions Committee of a veterinary college and ask yourself what you would look for in selecting the students most likely to succeed in veterinary medicine. There are probably three main points on which you would want to satisfy yourself when considering a student.

1. Are the prospect's academic skills and achievements sufficient to carry the professional curriculum?
2. Are his interests sincere, and are his background and familiarity with animals sufficient?
3. Are his health and personality traits compatible with the requirements of the profession?

Let us consider each of these points carefully. Now, while you are still in high school, is the ideal time to prepare yourself sufficiently so that when your application is presented, it will be stamped "Approved" by the Admissions Committee.

1. Academic achievements. While in high school, you should aim to get the best grades you can, to cover the proper subject matter, and to improve your communications skills. In judging an applicant's academic skill, both high school and pre-veterinary grades will be scrutinized. Grades

are an arbitrary, but fairly direct, way to determine whether the student can handle pre-veterinary and veterinary subjects. The student should stand in the upper two-fifths of his class, and the subjects taken should be those recommended for college preparatory work in the biological sciences, including chemistry, with a good background in English mathematics and physics.

Success in a profession depends greatly on being able to express and put your ideas across so that the ability to write and speak well is very important. The student who can converse with ease and confidence, who can read rapidly and write well, will find these skills greatly to his advantage. If you are wise, you will find out through your high school counselors and teachers how you rate in your skills of composition, comprehension, concentration, and reading. If you have any major deficiencies, correct them by extra work and special courses before you enter college. Once you enter the pre-veterinary college course, the grades you make will have to be high to meet with favor when reviewed by the admissions board.

In addition, the ability to use a typewriter is valuable and needed. Reports and manuscripts that are well typed when submitted mean a boost of as much as ten grade points over handwritten ones. Furthermore, since the veterinarian in practice may not always have a secretary, his ability to type health-examination records, committee reports, and correspondence will prove a big asset. In high school there may not be enough hours in the day to take a course in typing during the school year, but many students elect to enroll in a typing course during the summer session. Consider this; it is a very helpful skill to acquire.

In addition to high school, 3 to 4 years of college work

in pre-veterinary medicine are required before one can be considered for admission to a veterinary college. Here again, the grades you achieve will be the primary consideration in judging your academic ability. When you enter college, you will be assigned a counselor who will probably be a member of the veterinary faculty. With his help, plan your curriculum so that in these 3 to 4 years you can satisfactorily complete all of the required courses.

2. Sincere interest in and experience with animals. After the Chairman of the Admissions Committee is convinced that an applicant's academic skills are sufficient to carry him through a professional course, he will investigate whether the applicant's interest in veterinary medicine is well founded and lasting. From the standpoint of the applicant, his interest must be great enough to sustain him because it is difficult to shift to another line of study without loss of credits once the course is started. Then, too, consideration must be given to the great amount of money the university will invest in the student above the fee he will pay.

The student seldom realizes that the cost of his college education will be far greater, than the amount of money he pays in tuition and fees. Therefore, the school must have assurance that the student's interest is sincere. He will not only have to complete the course but he will be expected to serve the profession. The school will not have made a sound investment if the graduate leaves to go into a nonprofessional line of work upon completing his course, nor is it a good investment to choose a student only to have him withdraw in the middle of the course.

Sadder than this is that the student who quits has kept another deserving student out of the profession, because enrollment is limited by the physical facilities of each college. The number for which laboratory equipment and sink and desk space have been provided is limited. In the Appendix, following the list of veterinary colleges, there is a chart giving the number of students in each class at each veterinary college. If a place is vacated, it will remain vacant except for an occasional transfer of a student, which is rather rare.

If there is any danger that the applicant, either man or woman, may withdraw (with the consequence that taxpayers and others financing this education will not be repaid), that applicant should not be approved.

As far as a sincere interest in veterinary medicine is concerned, the applicant should have shown a genuine love for animals early in his formative years. He will probably have owned a variety of pets and, if raised on a farm or in a small community, he will probably have participated in 4-H club work, or joined the Future Farmers of America. Projects sponsored by these groups include raising horses, calves, pigs, sheep, dogs, chickens, rabbits, and guinea pigs. If the applicant lives in a more metropolitan area, he may have taken advantage of opportunities to participate in such activities as riding stable classes and nature study groups.

Youngsters fortunate enough to have been raised on a farm will learn what sanitary principles are necessary to raise healthy animals and to assure productive, healthy flocks and herds. This is fundamental knowledge. Most of us who grew up on farms took much of this training for granted. There is no substitute for "Science with Practice," which is the motto of Iowa State University, my alma mater. These fundamentals of herd management are the very things for which the veterinarian is responsible in his practice.

Any part-time and summer jobs the student has held will be scrutinized by the chairman of the admissions board to see whether they have been in the field of animal care. We have already discussed the desirability of working for a veterinarian in large- or small-animal practice. There may be many other opportunities for summer and after-school employment closely associated with animals. All drug manufacturing companies have experimental and research divisions, and they employ many trustworthy young men and women to assist with the tests and routines that are regularly performed in maintaining these animal colonies. Clinical laboratories at medical schools, hospitals, and research institutions all use animals in their work. Such opportunities for employment and experience should be investigated.

Students who like horses should not overlook an opportunity to learn about them. Riding stables are popular and available in most communities. Students who aspire to become veterinarians should learn to ride, groom, and care for horses. The art of horsemanship will be a very useful skill and will pay big dividends when horses are patients and horsemen are clients.

It is important to know whether the prospective veterinarian actually likes these tasks. For example, a young lady in our community prepared to be a secretary while she was in high school, but all through school she also had a horse of her own. After graduation, she continued to have an interest in horses, but obtained a position as a secretary. After working for a while, she became very discouraged because she did not like being confined indoors and begged her parents to allow her to quit. Finally, she resigned and took a job teaching horsemanship. At the end of her eight-hour day, she would come home and curry and exercise her own horse, then go to another riding academy where she taught horsemanship in the evening. On weekends, she and her brother, who also had a horse, attended horse shows. She worked longer hours at this than she had as a secretary, but she was happy, and the job did not seem like work at all. This kind of love and devotion for animals is what a veterinary student really needs to achieve success. With this sincere interest there is no doubt that he will be successful in any phase of the profession.

3. Health and personality. By the time the student has been in pre-veterinary training for a year or more, the members of the Admissions Committee board will have access to a fairly detailed record on these traits.

The health requirements for a veterinarian are rather demanding. Handling animals requires dexterity and at least average physical strength. The veterinarian must not only restrain the animals he is treating but also be agile enough to avoid being injured. Such clinical tasks as bleeding cattle from the jugular vein, delivering calves, or performing dentistry in the horse, require above-average physical strength and coördination. Such work rules out anyone with heart limitations, fainting spells, or severe physical disabilities or handicaps.

In pathology, good vision and color differentiation are essential. Good hearing is required to distinguish heart and intestinal sounds when making a differential diagnosis. Anyone prone to suffer from allergies or asthma should be discouraged because contact with the dander from hair of horses, cattle, cats, and dogs, and contact with various irritating bacteria make it impossible for those so afflicted to work without discomfort.

In considering an applicant from the standpoint of personality, it must be remembered that regardless of the special work followed by the veterinarian after graduation, selling services and advising animal owners about disease problems will be his most important functions. It would be difficult for the individual who does not like people, who is moody or uncoöperative, or who does not conform well to the rules of society to find a place in the profession. The candidates most likely to succeed are those who get along well with their classmates, who have high ideals, who are trustworthy, and whose appearance and manner are pleasing.

Pre-Veterinary Training

Now that we have looked at the problem of qualifying from the point of view of the Admissions Committee, let us consider pre-veterinary training. It is not necessary that the pre-veterinary medicine years be taken where you expect to take veterinary medicine. Students may take the pre-veterinary subjects at any college where they can meet the requirements in biology and other sciences.

Students with unusual ability in sports may be offered athletic scholarships and will want to accept. As a usual thing, it will be found that the work in a pre-professional school is too exacting to allow much time for a career in athletics. Those with unusual talent and desire for an athletic career have often elected to complete a bachelor's degree, and engage in athletics during that time. Then, when the eligibility has been exhausted, they will prepare for the professional school.

In choosing a school, the student must investigate the

geographical restrictions governing eligibility for each veterinary college. These agreements may limit your choice of school. As mentioned before, should you so choose, you may take pre-veterinary medicine at another university closer to home.

If you attend pre-veterinary school at the university where the veterinary college is located, start planning your campaign to get into veterinary college as soon as you arrive on campus. You should begin by acquainting yourself with the veterinary facilities so that you will recognize the different departments, such as anatomy, physiology, pathology, and clinics. An adviser is assigned to each freshman student; be sure that yours is a member of the veterinary faculty, for he can guide you in your pre-veterinary work. The chances are that he will be a member of the veterinary school Admissions Committee or at least closely associated with the men who are, so the impression you make on him is very important.

Most veterinary schools have pre-veterinary clubs sponsored by the veterinary students and faculty advisors, who want to get to know the new pre-veterinary students and help them become acclimated to the profession. Be alert for all of these opportunities and take full advantage of them. Not only will you gain, but this will be evidence of your interest in veterinary medicine.

I once knew a young woman from the East Coast who came to a Midwestern university to take pre-veterinary training. While in high school, she had worked in a veterinary hospital, and when she arrived at the university she found that she missed the animals very much. After a few days, she walked over to the veterinary school, quickly got acquainted, and asked the professor in charge of clinics if she could stay and watch. In a day or two, the clinician in charge found this young woman was picking up in the dispensary, washing instruments, and making herself useful. After three or four months of this, the director of clinics felt guilty about her doing all this work without compensation, and, because she was so valuable, he arranged a position for her with a small salary. For two years, she worked in the clinic whenever she had free hours. Finally, the time came when the pre-veterinary students were to be selected for admission to the veterinary college. She applied but, according to the rule among the deans, she was ineligible because she came from an Eastern state that had a veterinary school of its own. However, she had high grades and her impression on the Admissions Committee board was so favorable that the rules were waived and she was admitted.

If you love animals and are dedicated to their cause to the degree that you would rather care for them than do anything else, veterinary medicine is for you. Most of us in the profession feel this way, and once a young person makes up his or her mind that this is it, few ever leave. Who would want to do anything else? The rewards are worth all it takes.

Finances

Being admitted to college is only half the battle. The other, and probably the more frightening half, is financing an education. There is no doubt that paying one's way through college is a staggering task and only the wealthy can go in luxury. But most good students from families of low- and middle-income brackets can make it if a definite plan is developed and undertaken. The finances can be handled best by starting to provide the necessary funds for education several years in advance of time for college entrance.

The least expensive way to get the required years of preveterinary medicine, is to live at home and attend a state or locally supported college. Even then it may cost up to $1,000 a year or more.

In most universities full maintenance away from home, including tuition, room and board, and extra fees, reaches $2,000 to $8,000 per year, and a four-year course at a "prestige" college may cost as much as $5,000 to $10,000 per year. Although college expenses are now considered high, we may expect a continuing rise in costs at the rate of 4 to 5 per cent a year if present inflationary tendencies continue.

The old American tradition of working your way through college is out, as far as professional school is concerned. The increased academic demands leave little time for outside work. Many students combine "watch" jobs with studying and manage to earn part of their way. Typical employment would be a night watchman's job on a switchboard, in a generating station, or in an office or department store building.

The number of loans and scholarships available are increasing. However, most college administrators recommend that the student not plan to borrow or apply for a scholarship for at least the first year; he has to prove himself capable of handling college work before asking for assistance.

The student should therefore aim to have at least $3,500 to $10,000 saved to finance the first year without working. Then, if his college grades prove to be equal to the level necessary for admission to veterinary college, he can plan to seek enough outside work during the second year to finance one-fourth to one-half of the second year's expenses. A student can be expected to save from $600 to $1,000 from summer employment if he lives at home.

All colleges and universities offer a certain number of scholarships and loan funds to help students. There are increasing in number and amount as a result of growing contributions from alumni, from industry, and from other groups of Americans who are concerned about furthering higher education.

National Defense Act loans have become the main source of assistance for many students. These carry a small rate of interest (3 per cent), which does not start accruing until one year after graduation. Installment loans are offered by a number of finance and insurance companies. Some of these carry a reasonable rate of interest, whereas others are high. The rates should be investigated thoroughly.

A new idea is being tried in some veterinary colleges that provides continuous schooling without summer vacations. Once the student enters the professional school, he may complete his course in three years instead of four. The stepped-up program is known as the trimester system. However, this deprives the student of an opportunity to work at an outside job during summer vacations and earn part of his college expenses. The theory is that one year's time saved will more than compensate for the extra money that may have to be borrowed.

The American philosophy is that to get a good education you must want it, and that, if you want it, you should be willing to sacrifice and pay for it.

Veterinarians, almost invariably, have graduated in debt for at least part of their education. But the standing and potential income gained by a professional education is worth the effort and sacrifice necessary. The best advice for college financing is to start a savings program early with a definite plan to expand it continually over the years. This is a problem for the individual and his parents. For the bright, stable, conscientious student, there are usually enough possibilities available through private, local, university, and national sources to see him through.

CHAPTER V

Veterinarians in Practice

How to Enter Practice

Adapting oneself to the emergencies and challenges that constantly tax one's imagination and ingenuity in private practice offers the veterinary practitioner thrills and satisfactions that cannot be equaled elsewhere in the profession. In spite of hard work and long hours, practice holds more appeal for most of us than any other phase of veterinary medicine. Above all, each veterinary establishment, regardless of how big or small, is a public service to the community. The irregular hours and the need to be available at all times are probably the greatest disadvantages. Most veterinarians mind these very little, but such factors do require understanding and coöperation from his family. It seems that calls never come singly but in twos or threes, and schedules can never be maintained because unexpected interruptions occur day and night. But the excitement and anticipation are worth it.

Almost all veterinary graduates want to try practice first and by all means they should, even those planning a life work in research or teaching. Practice is the basis of our profession. Research and teaching must be designed for the benefit of practice; therefore, it is very difficult for a teacher or researcher to slant his activities in the direction of practice unless he has a firsthand knowledge of it.

Practice experience starts when the individual is still in school. During the summer and other vacation periods, many students work for veterinary practitioners. The experience acquired in this manner, either good or bad, will make a lasting impression, and, if the association is favorable, perhaps it will inspire the road to be followed by the student upon graduation. A summer job may even lead eventually to a partnership in practice.

How to start a practice is a serious consideration for the student. Taking care of animals successfully is quite a different thing from academic achievement in school. To make a correct diagnosis, help the animals, and satisfy the individual client require the kind of self-confidence that gives assurance to those who are depending upon you for service.

In school the training consists of learning skills in surgery, therapeutics, and medicine, and in practice these skills must be combined with judgment. The practitioner should know what is best for the patient, take into account the wishes of the owner, and be aware of his own abilities and limitations under given circumstances. It takes years of experience to learn to handle all of these factors correctly, and even then one cannot always do his work to the clients' satisfaction. The graduate should spend the first year with a seasoned practitioner in order to learn these things. The operation of a busy practice is major league performance and the young practitioner will need seasoning as does the rookie in the minor leagues before he goes to the majors.

At present, the veterinary profession has no internship requirement. Graduates are free to practice, but few feel confident enough to go it alone in the beginning. Since starting salaries are good, there is little reason why the graduate should not seek experience first. Then, after one or possibly two years, most veterinarians either obtain a practice of their own, become a partner in an established practice, or work on a salary-bonus arrangement where their effort and the value of the service they render are rewarded accordingly.

The ability and stamina of all individuals vary greatly. Some veterinarians work from dawn until dark, day in and day out, and thrive on it. Some others never become conditioned to the stresses and strains of such responsibilities. Each man has to make the adjustments and design his practice according to his individual talents, his physical make-up, his temperament, and what he wants to accomplish as a professional man. Most veterinarians graduate and start practice without knowing their own potentials or limitations. One veterinarian does well operating a large establishment with 15 or 20 employees, handles it competently, and is very successful, both professionally and financially. The next man may have equal professional ability but lack the executive know-how to run a successful business. The range of possibilities and the need for his services are such that he, too, can succeed and make a satisfactory living.

Over three-fourths, or 27,000, of the 35,000 veterinarians in the United States are in practice. Of these, 10,000 are in general practice, which means that they take care of larger animals (farm animals and horses) as well as small or pet animals. Then, 10,000 are in small-animal practice exclusively and about 2,000 limit their activities either to cattle, horses, swine, sheep, poultry, zoo animals, or fur-bearing animals.

General Practice

A general practitioner fulfills the needs of a rural community for veterinary service by treating all the farm animals as well as pet animals. The veterinarian responsible for such a practice usually spends about half of each day driving in the country making farm calls; the other half is spent at his office. The animals treated vary according to the geography, climate, land productivity, and the livestock common to the area.

In the New England and New York state area, for instance, a veterinarian will usually have his office in a small or medium-sized town. His establishment probably consists of an attractive small-animal hospital with a waiting room similar to that of any doctor's office. He has a receptionist who greets clients, answers the telephone, keeps records, and dispatches calls to the doctor while he is in the country. Like most practitioners, he keeps in touch with his office by means of a two-way radio. This keeps him aware of the activities in the office, as well as allows the receptionist to direct him to additional calls and to notify him of any emergencies.

The hospital usually consists of an examination room, operating room, drug room, and a ward or two with cages for pet animals; there also may be a large animal surgery and a few box stalls for hospitalizing large animals. His farm practice consists of caring for some chickens, a few riding horses, but principally dairy cattle. When he is not out on call or treating patients, the veterinarian develops and studies the X-rays he has taken in the course of his day's work, tests blood samples, and does other laboratory work. For example, brucellosis (contagious abortion of cattle) testing is routine. Dairy processing plants accept milk only from disease-free animals. Also, all breeding animals sold through public sale or transported across state lines must be free from brucellosis, and yearly testing is required. The veterinarian draws a sample of blood from a vein of the animal and tests this serum for reaction. He must test, record, and report on every dairy animal.

On the outskirts of all large cities there are dairy farms; this is known as the "milk shed" area. The milk is picked up daily from the farms and brought to large plants to be processed. Dairy herds today, although fewer, are much larger than ever before. The operating methods have become highly scientific and well organized, with greater milk production as the goal. Calves are vaccinated and cows are tested for brucellosis and tuberculosis at specified times. Artificial insemination and a controlled breeding program are practiced on most farms so that each female calf born is sired by a bull that transmits high productivity. The cows are examined regularly for pregnancy and mastitis as well as infectious diseases. Over the past several years, better feeding methods, a herd health program, better production blood lines, and improved sanitation methods have enabled dairies to increase production tremendously. The veterinarian not only answers service calls to treat sick animals, but he is the obstetrician, pediatrician, general practitioner, and herd health adviser. This work may be handled by the veterinarian on a retainer or contract basis.

Further south, along the Eastern Seaboard, a general

practice would be similar but would include the care of more horses, usually saddle horses and thoroughbreds, as well as some beef cattle.

In the Midwest, the veterinarian spends a large share of his time treating swine. Many farms are now stocked with "disease-free pigs." These pigs are born in a "pig hatchery" where there is a carefully maintained sanitation, breeding, and feeding program. When the pigs are weaned, at four to five weeks of age, they are sold to individual farmers who put them out on disease-free pastures. Hog houses are provided that have been scrupulously cleaned and are free of infectious swine diseases. With good husbandry methods and accelerated feeding programs, this kind of swine production puts the hogs on the market in the short time of five to six months.

In Nebraska, Colorado, the Dakotas, and Wyoming, the veterinarian conducts a ranch and feed-lot practice with cattle and sheep as his main interests. In these areas, the cattle herds are large and the ranches far apart. Some veterinarians of the range country fly their own planes in order to be able to make more calls and care for more herds. In the West, there may sometimes be as many as 10,000 beef animals either grazing or fattening in the feed lots. There are also many dairies in operation in the milk shed areas around the larger cities.

Ranches, like dairies, have consolidated and often thousands of animals are under the management of one company. Some companies both raise and fatten animals, particularly in the Denver area. Other companies raise the young animals and sell them to the corn-belt farmers of Indiana, Illinois, and Iowa for fattening. Again, the veterinarian's work here is often handled on a regular call basis as agreed upon between the veterinarian and the ranch manager.

The West Coast, from Washington to Southern California, has developed a great need for veterinarians. Irrigation has been a boon to agriculture in the Western Seaboard states, and they can now produce enough to feed the tremendously increased population in these areas. Los Angeles County in California has one of the largest cattle populations of any county in the world. Other counties in California, Washington, and Oregon are not far behind.

The demand for more veterinary service in the West has necessitated enlarging the veterinary college at Pullman, Washington, and brought about the founding of a veterinary school at the University of California. The school, at Davis, is on its way to becoming the largest veterinary school in the world.

Even the state of Alaska has need for veterinary service. Seventy-seven veterinarians are now located there; more will be added as the population grows. The state of Hawaii has proved to be a most delightful place to practice. Over 105 veterinarians are gainfully located there ministering to cattle, sheep, swine, mules, horses, and pet animals. Veterinarians help enforce Hawaii's rigid restrictions for importing animals. For example, dogs and cats must be isolated for 90 days before they can enter. This strict quarantine policy has kept the islands free of rabies.

Southwestern United States has always been cattle country, but with the growth of cities in Texas, Arizona, and New Mexico, there has been an increase in the number of horses, dairy cattle, and pet animals; thus, veterinary service has grown in proportion.

Florida and the Southeast at present form one of the

largest cattle-raising areas in the world. Formerly, the extremely hot, humid weather, coarse vegetation, and heavy infestation of parasites in the swamp lands made it virtually impossible for native cattle to grow and develop so that they could be raised profitably. This was overcome by introducing Brahma or Zebu cattle from India. These cattle are developed by nature to survive in a land with poor sanitation, a scarcity of food, and adverse weather conditions. They have stamina enough to maintain good flesh and withstand insects in the hot and sparsely cultivated areas of the South. Because the Brahma cattle are difficult to handle under range conditions because of their great strength and disregard for fences, they are crossed with beef breeds and domesticated while still retaining their hardiness and improved quality of meat. Now, with these hybrid cattle as much as one-seventh of our beef comes from the Southeast. Veterinary activity in Florida is no longer confined principally to the small-animal field, because now many veterinarians care for the cattle, horses, and other livestock that have been brought in as the conditions for them had improved.

Thus, we see that great strides have been made throughout the United States to improve livestock production. As the population grew in each area, the numbers of livestock increased. With this came also a desire for more companion animals. The added animal census in each area has brought greater demand for veterinary service and this will be true as long as the population continues to expand.

Today, a general practice is seldom conducted by one veterinarian whose office is a room in his house, as was the case a generation ago. The majority of practices are operated by at least two veterinarians. Frequently the practice is owned and operated by one man who hires a young man just out of school to assist him. The younger man moves on into a practice of his own as he completes his apprenticeship, and another graduate is hired to take his place. This creates a fine opportunity for the recent graduate to gain supervised experience. Sometimes he may even become the older man's associate or partner in practice.

Country practice is conducted on a twenty-four-hour call basis. Usually routine service calls are made between 8 A.M. and 5 P.M., but emergency calls come at all hours and somebody must be on hand to answer them. When two or more veterinarians are associated, these demands are divided so that each man will have some free time.

Primary assets for a general practitioner are good health, physical strength, and good coördination. He must be able to rope, tie, or otherwise restrain the animals he is to treat. He must be of fairly even temperament and competent enough to inspire confidence in the animals. With all the frustrations of a day's work he must develop a calm disposition so that his clients will learn to respect and trust his judgment.

He must be patient, observant, and keep good records, including case histories, a record of dosages given, and the results of his treatment. Good bookkeeping is also a requisite, both for regulatory reports required on all these animals and for accurate billing. For example, he takes and analyzes thousands of blood samples annually; these must be recorded accurately and without delay.

In addition to his home and automobile, the drugs, instruments, two-way radio, X-ray machine, and laboratory equipment essential to his practice would probably necessitate an investment of from $20,000 to $30,000. The facilities needed for the operation of a large-animal practice may vary greatly. The minimal requirement might be an office combined with the veterinarian's home, or the addition of one or two rooms at a cost of from $10,000 to $20,000. A hospital in a separate building apart from the home would probably range from $20,000 to $150,000, and, if the veterinary firm was large and employed two or three veterinarians, the cost of the facility might well exceed the latter figure.

What does the large-animal practitioner earn? The man who is well established, experienced, and capable of handling a large volume of work, will earn between $25,000 and $50,000 a year. The assistant veterinarian just out of school will start at around $25,000 a year plus car expense, and he can expect to have his income increase at a rate of $1,000 to $2,000 per year for the next five years. His advancement to the higher figures will be according to opportunities in a particular practice, how well he adapts himself to practice, and his individual abilities and skills. Success in any profession depends on the sum total of a man's attributes, his abilities, his skills, his work capacity, compatibility with people, his business sense, and the potential of the region; all are important. Financial prosperity is not the only major success. There is great reward in the knowledge that the work done has been truly helpful to patients and clients.

Equine Practice

Fifty years ago, the horse was the most important animal treated by the veterinarian. The majority of horses and mules used at that time were all important to agriculture, cartage, and military and private transportation. The introduction of motorized transportation and tractors forced the retirement of the draft and carriage horses. From 1920 until after the close of World War II there was a drastic yearly decline in the equine population. However, since World War II there has been a steady revival of interest in the horse, not as a beast of burden, but for racing, riding, and companionship. The popularity of race tracks, saddle clubs, and riding clubs, as well as ponies for children, has increased the demand to such a point that there are now an estimated 3 million horses and ponies in the United States.

The horse, whether at the track or for individual pleasure, has a great appeal for most people. On weekends and off-hours, an increasing number of Americans are spending time with them. Besides the thoroughbred, all classes of light horses are widely appreciated, from those used for pleasure riding along bridle paths to those used for skilled riding in polo and steeplechase racing. Youngsters start out on ponies and by stages graduate to larger animals. Fox hunting and steeplechasing provide places for the thoroughbred horses that are not fast enough for the race track.

The equine practitioner is concerned with the horses on stud and breeding farms, pleasure horses, and with those in training and racing. In the first type of practice, the veterinarian devotes time to treating reproductive difficulties in stallions and brood mares as well as caring for the foals and seeing that all of these horses are kept healthy.

The young thoroughbred race horse is put into training near the middle of his second year. Previous to this he has been taught to lead, pose, and be ridden. He has also become familiar with large crowds and the starting gate; he has been tested for speed. The standardbred has undergone similar training except that he has been taught to pull a cart, better known as a sulky. When a colt shows promise as a racer, he is slowly put in training. If the animal does not seem to have enough speed and its disposition is satisfactory, it may be converted to a steeplechase runner or a jumper.

Running horses, both thoroughbreds and standardbreds, require special attention, conditioning, and training to keep them racing. The usefulness of a running horse is only a few short years—usually one or two years and rarely more than five. A winning horse is capable of earning large sums of prize money, and the longer his performing ability can be preserved the more valuable he is. Care and training for these horses are very expensive, and thus it is a duty of the trainer and the veterinarian to keep the animals sound for as long as possible to return the owner's investment.

Illnesses of the running horse are of three types: traumatic, which is injury usually to the legs; contagious diseases, which for the most part are respiratory or influenza-like in type; and the colics, which stem from indigestion or faulty circulation to the intestinal tract.

A horse running at top speed carrying a man and saddle or pulling a man in a sulky is subjected to undue stresses and strains on the legs, which cause injuries to the bones, tendons, and ligaments. These injuries vary from minor sprains to severe untreatable fractures of the bones. The thoroughbreds that gallop and carry a rider injure the front legs usually, while the standardbred that pulls the sulky is more likely to injure the back legs. Treatment of these injuries consists first of radiographing the leg in order to make a diagnosis so that correct treatment can be prescribed; then rest, mild exercise, injections of cortisone, applications of heat or cold, and perhaps X-ray therapy are prescribed. In the case of some fractures, surgery may be performed. If the break occurs in one of the small bones, the pieces of bone that are chipped off are removed and the horse restored to racing service. If the injured animal has valuable blood lines and recovery is not complete, it may be retired to a breeding farm. Fracture of one of the main long bones of the leg still presents an often hopeless situation in which it is impossible to save the animal. In these instances, the horse is destroyed at the time the accident occurs.

All young horses are subject to respiratory viruses that cause pneumonia, sinusitis, and abscesses of the lymph nodes that drain the head and lungs. These infections can be very severe and take months to cure before training can be resumed. Antibiotics have been of help in controlling these infections.

Change of grain, hay, and water along with fatigue and stress are often responsible for digestive disturbances such as diarrhea and colic. When a horse is in abdominal distress, it will lie down and roll, kick, get up, and then throw itself on the ground. These signs are indicative of colic. The veterinarian gives drugs hypodermically and by mouth to relieve pain during such attacks.

Changes in circulation to the stomach and intestine will cause similar signs of colicky pain. A parasite, known as strongyloides, is a round worm that lives in the intestine. The larvae from this parasite migrate through the tissues during their life cycle. The wall of the arteries to the intestine is one of the tissues in which the larvae appear. Their presence in the vessels sometimes sets up such a reaction that circulation is reduced and tissues suffer from lack of oxygen and nutrition, causing severe pain. In rare instances, a major blood vessel will rupture, followed by death from hemorrhage. This parasite and a number of others have to be controlled. Regular fecal examinations are made to check for the presence of parasites. If they are found; the doctor then prescribes specific drugs, some of which are added to the food rations in dosages determined by the amount of infestation. These parasites live on the blood and body fluids, and the animal is "unthrifty" as a result. A heavily parasitized animal is never in top condition and seldom reaches its winning potential. Veterinarians are kept busy with the challenge of keeping the horses in good health as well as tending to their injuries.

The blood lines and genetics of thoroughbreds are of the utmost importance to the racing industry. When mares are bred and when colts are foaled witnesses certify the identity of the horses. Each horse is tatooed on the inside of the upper lip shortly after birth. By this he is identified with his pedigree, which denotes his ancestors and their records for generations.

Life insurance policies are carried on race horses. The more valuable ones are insured for several thousand dollars and a few for around a million. The value of a horse depends mostly on his winning potential and an owner has invested heavily in the animal by the time he is raised, trained, and conditioned for the track. Fatal injury would bring great financial loss.

When horses become unable to win, they are retired to riding stables if their ability and disposition are suitable. A select few that have superior track records and outstanding blood lines are retired to breeding farms to be used as sires and dams.

In addition to those doctors who treat horses at the track, three or four veterinarians are employed to guard the interests of the track owners and the state. Specifically, these men see that owners and trainers of horses abide by racing laws and the laws and regulations set forth by local, state, and federal government. These veterinarians examine the animals at the track to determine their fitness and soundness to run. All horses must be in good health and be free from lamenesses and unsightly blemishes. There are strict regulations controlling the use of drugs and special foods to stimulate a horse at the time of racing. In most instances, it is illegal for a horse to receive drugs either by injection or by mouth for a period of 72 hours before the time it is to race. Most drugs can be detected by testing the saliva and urine of the horse. The veterinarian checks specimens of all winning horses immediately after each race. The performance of the horses is monitored by movies and by the track veterinarians with field glasses to see that they are not lame or subjected to injury. If a horse becomes lame, it is declared unfit to race again until the lameness disappears.

Racing lasts for only a few weeks at each track and then the animals, the trainers, and the veterinarians move to another track. In the summer most of the racing is in such Northern states as Illinois, Michigan, New York, and New Jersey. In winter these same owners and trainers race their animals in Florida, Arizona, and California. Some of the same equine practitioners and veterinary track officials follow the horses to the various tracks. In order to do this, it is necessary that the veterinarian have a license to practice in each of the states where there is a major track.

The salaries and compensation received in equine practice are comparable to income from other phases of the profession. Those who make regular calls at the training barns and track stables are paid by the owners of the horses on an individual service-call basis. Those employed by the state or track are paid a salary at so much a day for their services.

Making service calls for racing animals does require some special equipment, most of which can be carried in the veterinarian's automobile. Some have trailers, which they move from track to track, containing laboratory equipment, X-ray developing tanks, and a portable X-ray.

Small-Animal Practice

After World War I, veterinarians in metropolitan areas recognized a growing demand for the care of pet animals. The family horse, cow, and chickens had gradually disappeared from the scene in urban areas and, because families liked animals about the place, pets were substituted. In this transition, each family was reduced to having only one or two pet animals, which became very precious to them. Good medical care was therefore demanded, and veterinarians who turned to give this their full attention soon realized that there were aspects of the field of small-animal practice that had not been explored. They discovered that both the dog and cat adapt well to anesthesia and to medical and surgical treatment, and that it was possible to perform delicate and complicated procedures safely. It was no longer necessary to destroy injured or sick animals. Broken bones could be set, tumors could be excised, and hemorrhages could be controlled.

Now almost half a century later, due to the expansion of urban living as well as to better veterinary medicine, the small animal population in the United States consists of approximately 40 million dogs, 40 million cats, and some 20 million other assorted species of animals and birds that are fed and cared for by an appreciative public.

An interesting and important sidelight is the economic value of the dog and cat. The small-animal population in this country provides a market for a sizable portion of our agricultural output and generates a volume of business and employment for our nation. Although many animals are fed table scraps, the dog and cat food industries annually process and sell over 3 billion pounds of pet food. The annual dollar volume of this rises well over 400 million dollars; of course, there is also an appreciable impact on the transportation industry that moves this food, as well as the steel and paper industries that furnish the tins and boxes to package it. It is estimated that a dog eats one-fourteenth as much food as a man does. On this basis, dogs alone consume as much food as is produced in all of the New England states, New York, Pennsylvania, Delaware, New Jersey, and Maryland. Without this outlet for agricultural products, our present problem of farm surpluses would be even more acute. Agricultural interests should be charitable to all phases of the pet industry when it comes to providing for veterinary schools.

The desire of the pet-owning public for preventive medical care, good diagnosis, treatment, and skillful surgery created the necessity for hospital facilities. By 1933, enough veterinarians were devoting full time to small-animal medicine for it to become a specialty and, in turn, for many small-animal hospitals to be built.

It was felt that an exchange of ideas was needed that would enable veterinarians to compare and improve their veterinary skills and methods as well as their small-animal facilities. As a result, the American Animal Hospital Association was formed in 1934. The objects of this association are stated in their constitution.

Section 1. To provide the best possible veterinary service and hospital facilities for the care and treatment of dogs, cats, and other pets, including caged birds.

Section 2. To advance the professional interests of veterinarians engaged in the hospitalization of small animals.

Section 3. To establish and maintain a high standard for the hospital, the equipment, the personnel, and the methods employed.

Section 4. To disseminate helpful information among owners of small animals to neutralize the ill effects of widely circulated misinformation, pertaining to the health of small animals and the treatment of their ailments.

Section 5. To coöperate with the section on small-animal practice of the American Veterinary Medical Association.

Section 6. To coöperate with our colleges in elevating the standards of veterinary education.

Section 7. To encourage progress in and coöperation between small-animal hospitals.

In addition to these objectives, the American Animal Hospital Association provides strict annual inspection of its member hospitals. Any hospital that fails to meet the requirements of humane, modern care is dropped from the roll. The Association, now over forty years old, has had a steady growth in membership, resulting in the greatly improved quality of veterinary service and facilities. As noted earlier, 10,000 veterinarians, of the 27,000 in practice, devote their time exclusively to small-animal care and, in addition, most large-animal practitioners take care of some pet animals.

Small-animal hospitals are now numerous in the suburbs

of large cities. Some are also found in the cities themselves, but restrictions imposed by apartment house owners have decreased the pet population in the multiple dwelling areas and the need for veterinary hospitals in the city has diminished accordingly. However, pets have increased markedly in areas of single family dwellings typical of the suburbs.

The size of hospitals varies from a small outpatient clinic, where no animals are kept overnight, to large hospitals with one hundred to two hundred individual compartments for animals. The large hospitals render a complete service and keep animals as long as desirable. They offer services of an outpatient clinic, laboratory, X-ray unit, operating room, and medical facilities. The average hospital has facilities for 25 to 50 animals. The number of veterinarians employed in these institutions varies with the conditions and type of practice, but on the average there are from one to four. There is also a staff of non-professional employees who feed and care for the animals under the doctor's direction.

The average veterinary hospital is equipped with an attractive waiting room where a receptionist greets the clients who come in or call by phone. She also keeps the books and records; if the hospital is large, two or three receptionists may be needed to carry the work load. The modern hospital is climate-controlled with regulated air-conditioning for coolness in summer and warmth in winter. Also, in order to avoid disturbing the neighbors with the nuisance of barking dogs, there are usually no windows and the exercise wards are enclosed and soundproofed.

The cost of building a hospital today is roughly from $50,000 to $150,000. It is usually estimated that ten to twenty-five hospital patients and the accompanying surgery, laboratory, treatment rooms, X-ray equipment, and ward space are sufficient to occupy the full time of one veterinarian.

When a new practice is started, naturally the volume of work is small. One veterinarian, with perhaps a lay assistant, is all the help that is needed. Such a practice is often started in a rented store building because the doctor's funds are limited at first. In converting a store, temporary partitions are adequate until the practice grows and the business warrants a more desirable facility. Then a new hospital is designed and built with all the rooms and conveniences necessary for efficient operation. It is well for the young graduate to remember that the American Animal Hospital Association maintains a service for aiding those veterinarians who want to obtain information on how to construct an animal hospital. Consult your local library for publications which describe in detail the most desirable floor plans, structures, and equipment.

As the practice grows, the director may hire non-professional assistants and, when justified, an assistant veterinarian. Here again, as in general practice, is an opportunity for the new graduate to serve an internship. The young person usually stays a year or two until enough experience is gained and enough capital is saved to buy an established practice, go into a partnership, or start a new practice. Undoubtedly, in a matter of a few years, organized internship and resident training for the veterinary graduate will be developed so that most graduates will take such training as part of their license requirement.

In choosing a location, one must always question the volume of work needed to provide an adequate income for a veterinarian and his family. Most practitioners located in a good growing suburban development will find that their practice increases substantially every year. It is difficult to estimate the amount of veterinary service that is needed by a community, but experience has taught us that a population of 35,000 will own enough animals to require the services of at least one veterinarian.

During the years of academic training, the veterinary student has very little time to gather other than professional experience. A doctor's skills in diagnosis, treatment, and surgery are fundamental for a successful practice, but he must also have the ability to handle people and finances.

The director of a practice must wear two hats: one as a professional man, and the other as a business executive. As a professional man, of course, he must see that the animals are adequately cared for; that diagnosis, treatments, and surgery are efficiently and skillfully executed; and that the hospital is kept clean and orderly.

As a businessman he must be an office manager, auditor, personnel director, purchasing agent, and, in a pinch, janitor. The American Animal Hospital Association Committee on Membership and Inspection found in a survey that the veterinary hospital director often needs help to improve his business methods and management. This is not surprising because veterinarians are not trained to be executives. The average small-animal hospital is not of sufficient size for it to be economically possible or practical to have a business manager. Therefore, the veterinarian must be responsible for seeing that charges are adequate, on a cost-accounting basis, that people pay their bills, and that there is sufficient income to pay himself, his employees, and his expenses. The bookkeeping system must be carefully worked out and accurately kept; income tax, withholding tax, unemployment compensation tax, real estate tax, workmen's compensation, and other such items must be paid promptly to the respective agencies. The employees, the building, the business, the patients, and the clients must all be protected by insurance. As purchasing agent, the veterinarian must see that supplies are ordered and paid for, and that food and drug inventories are kept current to avoid spoilage and waste; this is known as inventory control. Few professional people have had training in these business aspects and so the professional man must learn, with the help of a financial advisor, an auditor, and a lawyer, how to execute his office procedures adequately and efficiently.

The management aspect of practice is described in detail because so often young veterinary students and even graduates meet the real practice situation with consternation. I recall vividly one young man about to graduate from veterinary school who, having accompanied me and my two veterinary assistants for a few days as we attended the routine work of the hospital, confessed that he was disillusioned. He had envisioned the doctor on a lofty plane, attending only to complex diagnostic problems and complicated surgical procedures. He had not known that it is the large volume of repetitious vaccinations, minor injuries, and recurrent wormings and skin cases that keep a hospital going. Nor had he realized that there would be any problem in maintaining a smoothly running hospital, or that the director must assume supervision of all jobs from the maintenance man on up. He must even be willing to step in and add to his own work that of any employee who is absent or temporarily overworked.

The hospital director not only gains the benefit of his employee's abilities but also must tolerate his faults, inefficiencies, and idiosyncrasies. To some extent, the director also assumes the family problems of all the staff; if there is illness or trouble, he will find that the employee's family will lean heavily on him for advice and more often than not for financial assistance. In contemplating a practice, therefore, it must be realized that the most efficient operation is that conducted by the veterinarian and one lay assistant; each time an employee is added, whether lay or professional, the efficiency of the organization is lessened in proportion. Then it is the skill of good management that brings about the teamwork and coördination essential to success.

This simply means that the quality and promptness of the service, the orderliness of the building, the housekeeping, and the management in general are dependent upon how well the director's leadership and drive inspire coöperation in his employees. Some hospital directors can run a large practice with as many as twenty employees and keep them happy, contented, and hard-working, while another veterinarian has difficulty in maintaining a similar situation with two or three employees. The ability of each individual varies, and, as each veterinarian gains experience and is ready to assume the directorship of a hospital, he must weigh his aptitudes and desires and gear his own establishment accordingly.

Now, let us take a look at an average working day in a small-animal practice. The door of the reception room is open to admit patients for about ten hours each day. The hours maintained by the doctors vary with the community and with the preferences of the director. Usually the day starts at seven o'clock each morning, with an attendant in charge to admit animals as the clients drive by on their way to work. In most hospitals, the doctor arrives by seven-thirty or eight o'clock. In areas where there is seemingly no demand for this early morning service, it may be as late as nine or ten o'clock before patients are received. This is often the case if evening office hours are observed.

A doctor begins his day with a check of the patients. The ones admitted during the night or early morning are given attention first. The doctor acquaints himself with the attendant's record of the history of the patient's illness and learns whether the dog has vomited, had a bowel movement, or has eaten since its arrival. A temperature reading plus an examination of the patient will enable the doctor to make a preliminary diagnosis and lay out procedures, depending on what further observations are necessary. When the medical patients in the hospital have all been checked, those scheduled for surgery that day are given preoperative examination and medication. The doctor then gives his directions for the preparation of instruments, surgical packs, and the operating room. The doctor's assistants make these preparations while he sees his convalescing patients. Treatment, such as the administration of fluids and blood or changing of surgical dressings, is completed by the time the surgery schedule commences. In a two-man practice, the doctors usually alternate: while one performs surgery, the other tends to the office calls.

In a hospital, an average of two or three operations are performed daily. Some of these are relatively simple, such as trimming the ears of a boxer or schnauzer puppy or spaying a dog or cat. There are also more complicated tasks such as inserting a stainless steel pin in a fractured leg, amputating a mammary tumor, or removing a section of bowel that has been damaged by a foreign object the dog may have swallowed, such as a marble or a rubber ball.

Probably one of the most exciting procedures for the doctor and the members of the hospital staff is the Caesarian operation. After a female has been in labor for several hours and the doctor is unable to help her to whelp the puppies naturally, he must remove the young animals through a surgical opening made in the abdominal wall and into the uterus of the mother. Boston terriers and some other toy breeds often require Caesarian operations because of their small pelves as does any dog or cat that may have previously suffered a crushed pelvis, which makes natural birth impossible. There is a shared thrill of accomplishment when this is successful. Drying off and rubbing each pup until it gasps for that first breath with the cry typical of a newborn animal is a wonderful experience. The pups are put in an improvised cardboard crib on terry-cloth towels warmed with an electric heating pad on the bottom of the box. They are tended carefully for the first few hours until the mother has recovered sufficiently to care for and nurse them without help.

The only relatively quiet time at a hospital is from lunch time until three-thirty. This period is taken up with diagnostic work. For example, a dog with nausea and abdominal distress that was brought in during the morning may show signs of an intestinal obstruction. If the dog belongs to a family that has small children there is good probability that it may have eaten a small toy or other article. It must be determined whether the dog is sick from an ordinary stomach ache or if the condition is more serious. Such a patient is sedated and given barium by mouth; then an X-ray film is taken every thirty minutes to determine whether the barium solution passes through the intestinal tract or is obstructed at a certain point. Often an object like a rubber toy or a rubber baby nipple may be identified as the cause of vomiting. If a foreign object is identified on the film, the owner must be contacted for permission to remove the object without delay. In addition to the radiographs, this is the time of day when other laboratory procedures such as blood counts and urinalyses are done.

Shortly after three-thirty, mothers with their children just out of school begin to arrive. One of the pleasantest sights is a child receiving his treasured pet in the reception room; it is often hard to tell whether the child or the animal is happiest. From mid-afternoon until dinner time, the hospital personnel work at top speed, taking care of office calls and admitting and dismissing patients. Many hospitals close at six o'clock, while in others the doctors may alternate in keeping evening office hours.

The telephone is very important to every practice. It is the means by which the owner keeps in touch with the progress his pet is making, and at least one call a day can be expected about each patient. The doctor talks to the owner if the condition of the patient is critical, but in most instances the receptionist can give a progress report to the client. The receptionist is an important member of the staff. She, or he, must be a person with a pleasant voice who likes people and animals and who is not annoyed by the questions of animal owners. Telephone conversations tend to become routine to the one who answers the phone, but to the owner of the pet the call may be the most important one of the day. Clients resent having to talk to anyone who does not share their interest and concern. Probably the most successful practices are those that operate on an appointment basis both for seeing clients and for telephone conversations.

In all hospitals where animals, particularly surgical and medical patients, are kept overnight an attendant must be on duty around the clock to see that care is given when needed and that the doctor is called in case of hospital or outpatient emergencies. The American Animal Hospital Association requires that somebody be in or near the building at all times; the welfare of the animals must be the primary consideration.

Although much of the work of routine vaccinations, minor infections, and ear problems is repetitious, no day lacks interesting highlights nor is any day free of unusual problems. For those who love animals, who love and respect the dignity of life, this is work that is very satisfying.

As in general practice, those interested in small-animal practice ask the question, "What does the small-animal hospital director earn?" Again we say that his earnings will be substantially good. For the recent graduate without experience the starting salary is $300 to $400 per week, or $15,000 to $20,000 per year. This varies somewhat geographically and the advancement depends upon the man, the location, and the opportunity offered. However, as experience is gained and the individual assumes responsibility for his own work, the advancement and the income are commensurate with individual effort. In his own hospital a veterinarian's income will be greater.

Contributing to this will be his ability to sell needed services, the respect of the community for the image the veterinarian presents to his clientele, and what the veterinarian himself really wants out of life. If he wants above-average practice volume and income, if he wants a reputation for doing better than average work, then his work output and his willingness to satisfy clients must also be above average. Needless to say, his work week must be much more than an eight-hour day in a five-day week.

The income for a beginner who starts his own practice may be low at first, perhaps not more than a net of $400 or $900 a month, or less than $10,000 for that first year.

Growth is usually gradual but steady, and the beginner must be prepared to wait patiently until he becomes well enough known and established in the community for this to increase. The average net income is well worth waiting for, because it averages over $20,000 annually and there are a number of practices that yield in excess of $50,000 annually.

Zoo Practice

Zoo veterinarians have many fascinating stories to relate; unfortunately few of them have written much on the subject. There is one book, however, written by Dr. J. Y. Henderson and entitled "Circus Doctor" that makes wonderful reading. Here you can vicariously face such problems with Dr. Henderson as how to worm a bear and how to pull a lion's tooth.

Almost all cities have zoos and there are always one or two veterinarians who take an interest in this work. Some zoos employ a veterinarian full time, and at present the directors of three of our largest zoos in the U.S. are veterinarians—Chicago, Cleveland, and San Francisco.

The care of zoo animals offers unique opportunities for study of nutritional problems, breeding and obstetrics, dentistry and disease control, as well as medicine and surgery.

In "Circus Doctor" Dr. Henderson wrote of the failure to get elephants to breed in captivity, although it would be a boon to circuses if this could be done. Very recently, nation-wide coverage was given to the first birth of a baby elephant in captivity. There was graphic portrayal of the veterinarian's vigil and a discussion of some of the lessons learned, which may be helpful in getting other wild animals to reproduce in captivity. Because of the difficulties and expense of capturing and transporting wild animals, as well as the dangers of importing new diseases along with the animals, it would be well to learn how to provide optimum conditions for their reproduction. As civilization spreads, there is also the possibility that many species may become extinct if we do not learn how to preserve them.

Nutrition and reproduction are problems because we do not know enough about the native diet and behavior of wild animals and because it is difficult to provide adequate substitutes. It is even surmised that diet deficiency may be a contributing factor in reproduction problems. Much more study is needed in this field.

Disease control problems are similar to those the veterinarian meets in ministering to all other animal life. However, one unique factor is that when these wild animals are caged for exhibition they come in close proximity with people for the first time, and many of them contract human diseases to which they have no immunity. Tuberculosis, the top disease on the list, causes much illness and loss of animal life. Probably you have noticed that monkeys and chimps are often shielded from viewers by a wall of glass. This is to protect them from colds and other respiratory infections to which they are very susceptible.

Treating wild animals is extremely tricky because restraint is so essential. Tame as some may apparently become, none of these animals can be trusted to coöperate as domesticated animals do. The most recent progress has been the invention of a dart gun from which a pellet containing a tranquilizing agent can be shot. The animal is soon temporarily paralyzed and can be secured by the handlers so that the doctor is able to make an examination and complete his treatment. Anesthesia may then be successfully administered if any painful or lengthy procedure, such as pulling a tooth, must be performed.

A sign of the times is that zoos now feature domestic as well as exotic animals. To the city-bred children a good look at a cow may be as much of a novelty as a close-up of a kangaroo. One zoo I visited recently offered, for the nominal sum of ten cents, a nursing bottle full of milk that one could feed to the baby lambs. This proved so popular, with children and adults as well, that the zoo had to keep three sets of lambs and rotate them to prevent overfeeding.

Zoos provide an essential service in our civilization. They offer education as well as amusement and are enjoyed by millions of people every year. They also provide a means of preserving unique specimens of animal life. There is inspiration for artists, writers, and philosophers, as well as refreshment of spirit for all. Veterinarians who are attracted to this work find it most rewarding.

CHAPTER VI

Veterinarians in Federal Services

The federal government is the largest employer of veterinarians, with about 4,000 on its payroll. Government veterinarians are provided with attractive civil service ratings, assured regular advancement, and a substantial retirement and pension system. There is an exceptionally wide choice of positions, and advanced training is offered in each field.

The idea of a program for protecting the health of the nation's livestock began to develop shortly after the Civil War. For at least one hundred years prior to this, there had been costly outbreaks of diseases such as Texas fever, hog cholera, anthrax, pleuropneumonia, and tuberculosis, which killed thousands of head of livestock. Diseases transmissible from the animals also caused loss of human life. This was a devastating situation for a young nation. With both the livestock and human populations increasing, it became evident that the problem of the control and elimination of disease had grown beyond the point where any individual or local group could cope with it, and additional help was needed.

By 1884, Congress felt that, if animal diseases were to be controlled, a regular staff of veterinarians must be employed to police the activities of the livestock owners, shippers, processors, and importers. Accordingly, Congress passed legislation establishing a federal agency to prevent entry of diseased animals from foreign countries, and to suppress and eradicate animal disease.

The new agency was called the Bureau of Animal Industry of the U.S. Department of Agriculture. It grew and broadened its activities as America grew and developed new problems. The Bureau, or the B.A.I. as it was known for many years, began its work with the investigation of such diseases as bovine pleuropneumonia, Texas fever, hog cholera, and fowl cholera, and the pages of its history tell many fascinating stories of successful disease eradication and control. In 1890, meat inspection was made compulsory for all packing plants engaged in interstate shipment of meat and animal products.

As time went on, the veterinary activities of the federal government were expanded to include allied fields outside agriculture, and the name B.A.I. was no longer inclusive enough to cover all aspects of the work. Now these are known as the Federal Veterinary Services, and the Agriculture Branch has become known as the Agriculture Research Service, or A.R.S.

Agriculture Research Service

The annual budget of the Agriculture Research Service is approximately 75 million dollars, and it is larger than any of the other veterinary services. Under the A.R.S. are (1) the Meat Inspection Division, (2) the Animal Disease

Eradication Division, (3) the Animal Inspection and Quarantine Division, and (4) the Animal Disease and Parasite Research Division.

1. Meat Inspection Division

This division has the responsibility for the before-and-after inspection of over one million animals that are slaughtered annually in this country. This assures the American consumer that the meat bearing the "Inspected and Passed" stamp is clean, free from adulteration, and obtained from healthy animals, and that the labeling of meat and animal products is accurate and reliable. Veterinarians in this division are also responsible for the control of animal diseases, including those transmissible to man.

When the meat inspection law was passed, it was primarily to satisfy the demands of European countries that were buying meat from the United States. However, in 1906 a comprehensive law was passed and all U.S. meat packers shipping meat and meat products interstate as well as abroad became subject to inspection. These laws enhanced consumer confidence in the safety, wholesomeness, and accurate labeling of meat and other animal food products. Today, about 3,500 employees carry out the functions of the division of Meat Inspection in 1,334 establishments in 546 cities. Of these, 750 are veterinarians, 2,500 lay inspectors, 25 chemists, and the remainder clerical, administrative, and supporting personnel. This represents 80 per cent of all commercially produced meat in the United States. The other 20 per cent of the slaughtering establishments are under state and local supervision.

These activities at federally inspected plants are largely supported by tax appropriations from Congress. Besides inspecting meat for wholesomeness, government veterinarians are on the alert for any livestock epizoötics that they may find in any animal coming to market. The meat inspection services are principally engaged in the following activities:

1. Examining food animals, including cattle, calves, sheep, swine, goats, and horses, as they are brought to slaughter to see that they are healthy
2. Testing, through post-mortem examination, each carcass at the time of slaughter
3. Destruction of all diseased, unsound, and unwholesome meat and meat products
4. Supervising the preparation of meat and meat products
5. Preventing the use of harmful preservatives
6. Supervising the application of marks to meat and meat products to show that they are "U.S. Inspected and Passed."
7. Preventing the use of false and deceptive labeling of meat and meat products
8. Certifying meat and meat products for export
9. Inspecting meat and meat products offered for importation into the United States
10. Examining meat and meat products for government purchasing agents
11. Insuring accuracy and effectiveness of the inspection procedures
12. Supervising the manufacturing and labeling of butter
13. Guarding against residues in meat, such as pesticides, drugs, and biological products

14. Developing and determining acceptable methods for humane slaughter of animals

Besides the one hundred million animals slaughtered annually in the United States under Federal Meat Inspection, there are approximately a billion pounds of food of animal origin imported into the United States from 36 foreign countries. This all has to be inspected under federal supervision.

2. Animal Disease Eradication Division

The Animal Disease Eradication Division was established in 1884. Its chief function is to prevent the introduction of any disease into the United States and to suppress the diseases that plague livestock nationally. Such activity is usually the joint effort of individual animal owners, veterinarians, and the state and federal governments. The federal government depends on the private veterinary practitioner to participate as a part-time employee to do the testing and to furnish required reports. Full-time federally employed veterinarians are responsible for the interstate and import inspection work. With the coöperative efforts of all these veterinarians, foot-and-mouth disease has been eradicated from the United States nine times and on many occasions during the past thirty years it has been prevented from gaining entrance.

In 1929, it was discovered that a peculiar disease causing fever blister lesions of the feet and mouth was affecting the swine and cattle in certain areas of California. Swine so affected refused to eat, lost weight, and did not fatten for the market. Dairy cattle developed ulcers on the udder, teats, tongue, and feet, and milk production decreased. The farmers sought help, and the veterinarians, seeing this disease for the first time, were puzzled as to what is was. Federal veterinarians were finally called in for consultation, and their tests showed that the condition was the dread foot-and-mouth disease. Its source was a mystery because this disease had occurred in America only eight times since 1870, and our country had been free of it for many years. Investigators started to trace the cause of the outbreak. After much sleuthing, it was discovered that meat scraps in the garbage taken from a foreign ship harbored the virus. For years it had been customary for hog feeders to pick up the garbage from ships that were in port and from restaurants for feeding their swine. Some hogs fed with this garbage became infected and from there the disease spread to other feed lots and to dairies. When foot-and-mouth disease was positively diagnosed, the infected areas were immediately quarantined and all cloven-footed animals, which includes cattle, sheep, goats, deer, and swine, were killed and buried. Laws were immediately passed that all incoming ships must dump their garbage in the sea beyond the twelve-mile limit.

I can recall as a student in veterinary school the discussions about this and the way some journalists dramatized the horrors of the drastic measures used to control the disease. Big pits were dug and animals were driven into these, shot, and then covered over with lime and a layer of dirt. The money spent to compensate the farmers for their animals and to finance this operation, and the waste of meat, seemed great at the time. However, it amounted to very little compared with the money other countries have spent trying to control the disease with vaccine and isolation, nor did it take into account the untold suffering and death that would have struck down a far greater number of animals affected with the disease if such drastic measures had not been taken.

These methods were severe, to be sure, but very practical. Only three nations—the United States, Canada, and Australia—have taken steps to kill all infected animals and thus to eliminate completely the virus of foot-and-mouth disease. Other countries cannot do this because their meat supply is so limited that killing infected animals would bring both bankruptcy to the countries and starvation to the population. They treat the infected animals.

Brucellosis is one of the major diseases of breeding cattle and it also stands high on the list of diseases transmissible from animals to man. A state and federal brucellosis eradication program, under way since 1934, is successfully reducing the incidence of this disease. The program consists of wide-scale vaccination of calves and a follow-up blood testing of adult animals. This work is supervised by federal and state veterinarians supported financially by the federal and state governments. Local veterinarians vaccinate and test the animals.

Bovine tuberculosis, which is also transmissible to man, is still found in some herds of cattle in the United States, although its incidence in both animals and man has been sharply reduced. There is a testing program for tuberculosis, similar to the one for brucellosis, which operates under the direction of the federal and state Animal Disease Eradication Division and the same local veterinarians participate. Animals are tested by injecting two drops of tuberculin solution under the skin of the animal. If the animal has tuberculosis, a swelling occurs at the site of the injection within 72 hours. Animals reacting to this test are condemned and destroyed. The owners of condemned cattle are compensated in part for their loss by indemnity payments from state and federal sources.

This program was initiated in 1927 and precipitated the "Cow War." You may not have studied about this in American History, but to the legislators, farmers, National Guardsmen, and veterinarians of Iowa this was a very important issue from 1927 until 1935. At that time, as many as 5 per cent of the breeding cattle in the Midwestern states were affected with bovine tuberculosis; human tuberculosis was contracted by drinking infected milk. Various groups of people interested in protecting the health of human beings and producing healthy livestock banded together and urged that cattle with tuberculosis be eliminated.

In 1932, the nation was in the midst of the Depression; cattle were cheap, the Midwest was suffering from a serious drought; and there was not enough feed for all the animals. Thus, it seemed to be an ideal time to destroy the cattle that reacted positively to the tuberculosis test. In accordance with this thinking, Iowa, as well as many other states, passed laws requiring the compulsory periodic testing of all breeding cattle and the immediate destruction of all that showed positive reactions. The federal government agreed to pay one-half of the fee for testing and one-half of the indemnity for infected animals; the state agreed to pay the other half.

In some of the Midwestern states, particularly Iowa, there was considerable opposition to the "Test and Slaughter" program. Many farmers did not want their cattle tested because the test was comparatively new and many old wives' tales and myths developed among farmers and ignorant folks regarding its harmful effects upon animals that had no disease. It was rumored that the animals, when tested, would die or lose their tails, become cripples, or abort their calves. The opposition bought radio time, held mass meetings, and printed volumes of handbills denouncing the program. Sometimes at meetings veterinarians were called in to explain the tests, but often the fanatical opposition was so loud and rude that many meetings ended in fist fights and local police officers had to quiet angered mobs. Cattle owners worried so much for fear of bad effects of the test that they banded together, threw up road blocks, and guarded their animals with shotguns to stop veterinarians from coming on their farms to test the cattle. The situation got so far out of hand in at least three counties of Iowa that the National Guard had to be activated; squads of soldiers accompanied veterinarians to farms to round up cattle and test them.

Finally, the testing was completed for the entire state. When the farmers realized that their cattle did not suffer, that the testing program promoted better health for their herds, as well as for the people who drank milk, the objections died down and there has been no more trouble since. But making the first tests was a costly and exciting experience for those who participated. In the beginning, one animal in every twenty was found to be infected; today, following repeated testing, the incidence is less than one in five hundred and many counties are entirely free of bovine tuberculosis.

The Animal Disease Eradication Division also has charge of the interstate shipment of livestock and the inspection and control of animals passing through public stockyards. The inspectors in this division also enforce the 28-hour law, which provides that all animals being transported cannot be confined in a truck or stockcar for any longer than 28 hours without being unloaded for exercise, rest, water, and feed.

3. Animal Inspection and Quarantine Division

The Animal Inspection and Quarantine Division encompasses two programs. The first involves the inspection and quarantine of imported animals and their by-products. The other includes the control of serums and vaccines for animals.

The importance of the Animal Inspection and Quarantine Division is probably best summed up by Col. Fred D. Maurer of the United States Army Veterinary Corps. He says, "Several infectious diseases of food-producing livestock have recently shown a remarkable ability to spread to previously uninfected countries. Although contagious diseases have always moved with their hosts and vectors, modern transportation has greatly increased the flow of trade and travelers between formerly remote regions of the world. Thousands of ships with fresh and frozen meat in their galleys and often with animals and animal products in their cargo enter foreign ports daily. Animal products in passenger baggage present a special hazard. In one year recently, U.S. port authorities confiscated 24,000 pounds of meat in small packages from the baggage of nearly that many people entering American ports. More animals, both domestic and wild, are now moved by air than by ship. Aircraft land at innumerable inland ports, often close to domestic livestock areas. Several of the world's most destructive livestock diseases have taken advantage of these opportunities to spread. This is especially true of the insect-borne virus disease.

"Blue tongue of sheep and cattle is typical of these diseases. . . . Since the fall of 1959, African horse sickness has spread from the historically enzoötic areas of Africa to ten countries of the Near East and Southeast Asia, causing an estimated loss of 300,000 horses, mules, and donkeys. . . . African swine fever, which has long prevented the commercial raising of swine in much of Africa, has spread to Portugal and Spain. Since 1957, it has led to the death of an estimated many thousand head of swine in those two countries and is threatening the meat supply of all Europe. This disease is clinically similar to American hog cholera. . . .

"United States food surpluses are unique in this world, but we do not have any significant surplus of animal products. Much of the world is short of animal protein, especially at a price the lowest income groups can pay. The presence of contagious disease in livestock-producing countries has long prevented trade with food-deficient countries which would gladly exchange finished goods for disease-free animal products. The economic burden imposed on succeeding generations by loss of food and trade from animal disease has been a major handicap to the development of many countries. Non-industrial, agrarian countries with potential food surpluses must be able to engage their food products in international trade if they and the food-deficient industrial countries are to prosper. Economic survival is essential to political stability.

"As the world's population grows and more people compete for food from the limited land areas, loss from animal disease and handicaps to the distribution of food will become even more intolerable.

"We learned long ago that it is in the common interest to eliminate cases of smallpox from a community, even if it must be done at public expense. It is now equally apparent that the presence of these animal diseases anywhere poses a threat to the food supply and the economy of all countries."

Animal import quarantine regulations cover cattle, horses, sheep, swine, and exhibition animals for zoos. These regulations also control the use and disposal of related materials such as meats, bones, blood, glands, manure, hides, and skins. Many of these products are imported for use in clothing, leather goods, feed, medicine, and fertilizers. Annually some 1,150,000 animals and 12,500 birds are inspected for import, and the amount of related materials used runs into thousands of tons. The work is conducted by 35 veterinarians and about 100 lay assistants. Quarantine stations are maintained at all U.S. ports of entry.

The officials of the Animal Inspection and Quarantine Division view with concern the luggage of tourists returning from foreign countries. Each year thousands of Americans visit relatives abroad and they are often given gifts of homemade sausage or cheese. Most of these products are prepared without cooking and could easily carry bacteria or viruses of a large number of diseases which are common in a foreign country but have been eliminated in the United States. It is irritating and disappointing for returning citizens to have to give up a remembrance from their foreign relatives, but one only has to remember the costly outbreaks of bovine pleuropneumonia and foot-and-mouth disease to realize that the risks are so great that these stringent measures are necessary.

The division also handles the licensing and inspection of veterinary biologics produced in the United States. This control work helps to insure the American stockman and poultryman of safe, pure, and effective products for their animals. Veterinarians are stationed at the various manufacturing plants to oversee and inspect the production of serums and vaccines.

4. The Animal Disease and Parasite Research Division

The Animal Disease and Parasite Research Division of the Federal Veterinary Services was officially started in 1954. This division has developed research programs in the fields of infectious and parasitic diseases. The work is conducted at three principal laboratories: the Parasitological Laboratory at Beltsville, Md.; the National Animal Disease Laboratory at Ames, Iowa; and the Plum Island Animal Disease Laboratory at Greenport, Long Island, N.Y. In addition, there are twelve field stations located at different points over the United States as well as laboratories in Kenya, East Africa; Fairbright, England; and Compton, England. The United States also has coöperative agreements with the Netherlands and Denmark.

Studies are continually being made on viruses, rickettsia, bacteria, fungi, and parasites with specific attention to tuberculosis, orithocosis, leptospirosis, swine erysipelas, brucellosis, and salmonellosis. Some of the non-infectious diseases include bloat in ruminants, livestock poisoning by plants, radioactive fallout contamination, and the effects of nuclear fission on meat, milk, butter, and leather.

These laboratories employ some of the best veterinary scientists in America today. The young veterinarian in search of new fields that offer exceptional opportunities for training would do well to explore the opportunities offered in research by the Animal Disease and Parasite Research Division. The National Animal Disease Laboratory at Ames, Iowa, for example, is located near the campus of the College of Veterinary Medicine at Iowa State University. The directors are seeking the services of young veterinarians and arrangements have been made with the University for on-the-job training programs whereby the student can receive graduate training at the same time he is working and gaining experience at the laboratory. His work at the laboratory can be planned so that it serves as the thesis material for his advanced degrees.

Public Health

Since 1920, veterinarians have been employed in health and sanitation activities on local, state, and national levels. Until 1950, they served principally as milk specialists, because milk is one of the food products that must be closely watched; diseases such as typhoid, scarlet fever, diphtheria, tuberculosis, and brucellosis are readily spread through contaminated milk. Much of the pioneer work in developing ordinances that raised the standard of sanitation and the quality of milk in the milk shed areas of most of the large cities was performed by veterinarians.

On a local level, approximately 1,200 veterinarians in the United States are employed in various capacities by city and county governments. In each community health and sanitation problems are usually handled by a committee of interested citizens. The members are ordinarily local volunteers, including physicians, dentists, local sanitary engineers, and veterinarians. The administration of the department is often conducted by a hired employee such as a police or sanitary officer. In areas with special problems like rabies control a program may be under the direct administration of a locally employed and commissioned veterinarian.

On the state level, thirty states have veterinary public

health programs. To assist the national program, each state has public health officers, including veterinarians, whose primary responsibility is that of controlling diseases transmissible from animals to man. They investigate such disease problems as outbreaks of leptospirosis, blastomycosis, histoplasmosis, scarlet fever, and brucellosis. These local and state organizations can, and often do, call upon the U.S. Public Health Service for assistance and advice.

In 1942, the U.S. Public Health Service commissioned veterinarians to serve as sanitarians during the war. In 1947, the U.S. Public Health Service created a Veterinary Section, which is a part of its regular corps and offers attractive commissions to veterinarians. Since 1950, as part of an expansion program, the PHS has employed veterinarians in comparative cardiology, cancer research, air pollution research, and radiological health. There are now approximately seventy-five veterinary officers on duty.

The U.S. Public Health Service engages in research, training, and consultation. Research ranges from the investigation of new infectious agents to the development of methods for improved diagnostic techniques. Training activities include holding regularly scheduled courses for veterinarians and other health officers in laboratory and field phases of disease control, preparing and publishing manuals and pamphlets, producing audio-visual aids such as motion pictures, and holding regional training conferences to disseminate knowledge about infectious diseases. Consultation is given to state or local officials who request assistance in solving disease problems. Technical aid is made available to curb disease outbreaks and to develop long-range control programs. For example, such coöperative programs have lowered the total number of rabies cases in the United

States 60 per cent in the last fifteen years, and at the same time the number of human cases have been reduced from twenty-two to two per year.

Since 1959, the U.S. Public Health Service has sponsored a World Health Organization, which is designed to strengthen the area of comparative medicine and public health. Veterinary aspects of world health must be freely discussed and understood on an international scale if they are to be solved.

The types of Public Health Service assignments available to veterinarians were listed in a recent announcement as follows:

> Numerous opportunities in field investigations, research, and public health are available for veterinarians in the Public Health Service throughout the United States and overseas.
>
> *Field investigation of the zoönoses:* Investigations are conducted of those animal diseases transmissible to man (i.e., rabies, leptospirosis, psittacosis, and encephalitis). In areas where these diseases are enzoötic, Public Health Service field stations offer varied opportunities for training and experience in their ecology, epidemiology, and control.
>
> *Public Health:* Service veterinarians act either as consultants or active participants coöperating with local health authorities in demonstrating new methods of improving public health, controlling disease, and fighting epidemics.
>
> *Research:* The National Institutes of Health (Bethesda, Maryland), the Communicable Disease Center (At-

lanta, Georgia), the Arctic Health Research Center (Anchorage, Alaska), and the Division of Occupational Health (Public Health Service Headquarters, Washington, D.C.), provide research opportunities in many aspects of medicine and science. Research is also carried on in Public Health Service field stations throughout the United States.

To qualify, the applicant must have some professional experience in addition to his veterinary degree and must pass an examination. Promotions, compensation, and retirement pay are comparable with military assignments. Active duty as a commissioned officer in the Public Health Service satisfies Selective Service obligations.

As of 1980 the beginning salary varies from about $18,-000 for veterinarians with limited experience to about $22,-000 for those with additional training and experience. There are liberal salary raises. Retirement pay after thirty years of service, or at the age of sixty-four, is three-fourths of your annual basic pay at time of retirement. Twenty-year retirement is also possible.

Of interest to the veterinary student are the Public Health training programs in technical skills for the professional student who wants a career in Public Health. The summer training program not only carries an attractive salary for vacation-time duty, but the trainee is placed in an interesting type of work and gains valuable experience in his field.

Opportunities and needs are increasing for veterinary surveillance, research, control, consultation, and training programs on various phases of public health problems in government, industry, educational institutions, and private agencies.

Veterinary Medical Branch of the Food and Drug Administration

In 1906, Congress passed the original Pure Food and Drug Act, which was amended in 1938. Since 1953, the job of enforcing it has been up to the Department of Health, Education, and Welfare. In this vital area its regulatory agency, the Food and Drug Administration, which was formerly a part of the Department of Agriculture, is responsible for the ultimate protection of human health. The Veterinary Medical Branch, which is one of five branches of the FDA, is directly responsible for the safety and efficacy of drugs, devices, and medicated foods which are intended for use for livestock and poultry. The products covered by this branch amount to over 160 million dollars per year.

The veterinarian's responsibility is to see that the drugs are pure, wholesome, safe to use, made under sanitary conditions, and truthfully labeled. All new veterinary drugs must be submitted for testing before they can be marketed. The companies must show positive evidence that the product will cause no harmful effects and that it is labeled properly. When drugs are to be used for treating food-producing animals, it must be further substantiated that the residues, if any, left in the animal's body or released in milk or eggs, will not be harmful in any way to the consumer.

To give an illustration of the complexities that arise in modern medicine, many drugs now given to dairy cows for various ailments may be secreted in the milk. Therefore, the milk from a cow receiving a dose of antibiotics cannot be sold; furthermore, not until 72 hours after the use of the drugs has been discontinued can that cow's milk be marketed. Another example is that sex hormones, primarily estrogens, are often given to cattle and poultry to hasten fattening and tenderize the meat. The amount is rigidly controlled by the Veterinary Medical Branch because there is some residue of these hormones in the meat. If this were not regulated, it would be possible to produce sex changes in human beings who consumed the meat.

In the past few years, medicated feeds for animals have come into existence, particularly in the poultry industry; these too must be continually checked. These advances in modern feeding enable us to raise healthier, fatter animals in a shorter time, which is a great economic advantage to all concerned, but there is an element of risk that must be kept under constant surveillance.

The Food and Drug Administration is also concerned with radioactive fallout and foods contaminated by radiation. As our living grows more complicated with the products of science, there is no doubt that the FDA will have to grow to meet the needs of an expanding scientific world. This means more job opportunities and new avenues of service for those trained in this field.

Fish and Wildlife Service

Through the Department of the Interior, our national park system has made great effort and spent considerable money to preserve the wildlife that is left in this country. Disease is one of the most important factors influencing wild animal population levels. These animals and herds, like the domesticated ones, often become infested with parasites and suffer from a variety of infectious diseases. For example, large numbers of squirrels, waterfowl, and quail have been known to die from blood parasites. Hookworms affect seals, gizzard worms infest Canadian geese, and rabbits, raccoons, squirrels, and foxes are susceptible to a variety of virus diseases.

At least a hundred diseases that affect wild animals and birds can be transmitted between man and animals; therefore, health in animals is directly related to human health. In certain diseases, such as rabies, wild animals serve as the reservoirs or vectors. Foxes, skunks, and bats have been responsible for numerous outbreaks of rabies by transmitting the virus to dogs, horses, and cattle. The fact that it is impossible to round up and vaccinate these wild animals makes the control of the disease very difficult. Rodents are also known to be carriers of encephalomyelitis, leptospirosis, and such mycotic infections as coccidioidomycosis, histoplasmosis, and ringworm. Other transmissible diseases affecting wild animals are spotted fever, relapsing fever, tularemia, Q fever, and toxoplasmosis. Man likes to be close to wildlife and therefore it is necessary to see that he does not infect the wild animals and make it possible for them, in turn, to infect other men.

Few wild animals breed, reproduce, mother their young, or thrive except in seclusion. When natural foods and environment become exhausted, man must provide substitutes for these if the species is to be preserved. Veterinarians and wildlife experts continually strive to learn more about the habits and nutrition essential to the good health and preservation of wild animals.

Take one example of the problems they work with. In northwestern California, western Oregon, and southwestern Washington, dogs, foxes, and coyotes were dying of a disease known as salmon poisoning. The disease was known to the Indians and to the early settlers who gave the disease its name. Along about 1920 when the dogs of many sportsmen became ill and died, a general alarm was sent out for help. The story was always about the same: A week or ten days after the family had been on a successful salmon fishing trip the dog who was the household pet became ill and died. As was customary after arriving home, the fish were cleaned and the entrails and heads were discarded. Commonly, neighborhood dogs managed to invade the garbage and to eat some of the refuse. After a week or so, the dog would start to run a fever, lose its appetite, and become markedly depressed. In a few more days, the temperature would go up to 104 to 107 degrees and the dog would become very ill. Within a few more days, it would lose weight very rapidly, become so emaciated that only skin and bones were left. Within ten days, the animal would be so weak it would die. Besides the dogs that died, carcasses of foxes and coyotes were also found near streams and the Pacific Ocean. The losses in these animals became alarming.

The Wild Life Fish and Game Commission called in veterinarians for assistance. After some research on the problem, the complete story of the disease and its life cycle was gradually pieced together. It was found that salmon carry the eggs of flukes, which are small worms. These eggs are eaten by the dog, fox, or coyote, and hatch out into little cysts in the intestinal wall. The flukes are thought to carry a virus or some other infectious agent that is poisonous to these animals. The combination of the fluke plus the disease the fluke carried causes this fatal disease in such animals. When the flukes and cysts are passed from the body of the animal during its illness, they are eaten by snails. The infected snails go to the streams and rivers and eventually back to the ocean where they come in contact with the salmon and thus the cycle is completed. Not all of the problems connected with salmon poisoning have yet been solved, but treatment with antibiotics can now save most animals if drugs are given adequately.

The main laboratories for such study are located at the Communicable Disease Center at Atlanta, Georgia, and at Rocky Mountain Laboratory at Hamilton, Montana. This is a challenging and exciting career for the veterinarian who is a naturalist.

CHAPTER VII

Veterinarians in Teaching and Research

It is doubtful whether students ever start veterinary school with the intention of becoming teachers. The primary motivation for entering veterinary medicine is the desire to practice, treat, and care for animals. However, in the course of gaining a medical education new horizons are glimpsed, and some students find their interests taking a more analytical bent.

It is those students who are not satisfied to learn only what a disease is who demand more study. They develop an insatiable desire to know the answers to all the *whys* about a lesion or a disease, and through graduate study they become the new generation of research scientists and teachers.

It is a natural trait to want to teach others as one becomes proficient in any field; thus, there is an affinity between research and teaching. As insight and knowledge are gained, one has a desire to share this learning. Those in research always have a good grasp of the fundamentals to instruct and often the spark to inspire those who study under them.

Though the primary reason for the existence of a veterinary college is to train and graduate men and women who will be capable doctors, the veterinary school must always be a research center. Therefore, it is difficult to separate the teaching and research functions because they are so interrelated. Let us, however, give consideration first to the academic functions of a veterinary school and its faculty members. Each school is headed by a dean who is a veterinarian, usually with an additional degree of Ph.D., whose responsibilities are similar to those of the president of a company. The dean directs the activities of the school and is responsible for the curriculum, the staff, the students, and the budget. He represents the school and its interests in the university councils, before the agricultural interests of the state, to its alumni, and before state and national veterinary groups and associations. Deans carry great responsibility, and, quite fittingly, among them are some of the finest and most honored men in our profession.

Most of the veterinary colleges have five major departments—anatomy, physiology and pharmacology, pathology, microbiology and public health, and finally the medical and surgery department which also directs the clinics. Each department head holds the rank of professor, and there may be one or two other professors in each department along with one or two associate professors and two or more assistant professors. Below them in rank are the instructors. Graduate students are not considered part of the faculty, although they may do some teaching, particularly in laboratories and clinics.

The department head, whose administrative position is comparable to that of a vice-president of a company, directs both the teaching and the research in his specialty. It usually takes about fifteen years of teaching and advanced study to attain this status on a college faculty, just as it takes about that same length of time to become a vice-president of a company or a partner in a law firm.

The graduate student who is attracted to academic work is sought out and cultivated by veterinary faculties because teachers and others with advanced training are in demand. Thirteen new veterinary colleges have opened since World War II. This, plus accelerated research programs in federal and commercial organizations, has created a great need for trained veterinarians.

To qualify for a position as instructor, one need not always have a master's degree, but it is usually a condition of employment that it will be attained within an agreed period of a year or two. The instructor's schedule will be planned to allow for his own class and thesis work as a graduate student. As veterinarians in academic positions progress up the scale, it is incumbent upon them to continue their education. Most of them obtain an M.S. and many attain a Ph.D. Most universities allow for a sabbatical year, the traditional one year off after each seven years of teaching on a university faculty, which, it is hoped, will be used for study. Also in fields such as veterinary pathology special preparation leads to qualifying for Boards of the American College of Veterinary Pathology. As in human medicine, passing one's board examinations is a mark of such proficiency in that special field that it is often considered to be equivalent to a Ph.D.

The salary scale in academic work has increased markedly since World War II, but so has the cost of living. Today, roughly speaking, an instructor begins at $10,000 to $14,000 a year and progresses from there. The range for assistant professors is about $15,000 to $25,000, associate professors $20,000 to $30,000, professors $25,000 to $40,000, and deans $40,000 and above. In today's competitive economic situation, these salaries do not always sound glamorous. Actually, they permit a good living in keeping with the standards of one's colleagues in university circles.

There are many other assets that carry more weight in a life than those measured by monetary standards. A young professor loves teaching and research for their own sake, and he enjoys conferring with young people; he appreciates the opportunity to carry on investigation in his particular specialty, and enjoys life in the intellectually and spiritually stimulating atmosphere of a university. There is also the advantage of raising one's children in this desirable cultural climate.

Now, let us consider the research activities of the schools of veterinary medicine. Besides teaching, all departments carry on some research projects. Research is of two types—basic and applied. Perhaps it would be appropriate here to go into this distinction. Basic research connotes investigation of a scientific question or problem simply to find the answers, without concern for the application of the results. This is sometimes referred to as "pure research" and is in keeping with the traditional professor and his ivory tower approach. It refers to the tedious compilation of data in little understood areas simply to find out more about all the facts contributing to any specific phenomenon without concern about the usefulness of the results. It is not to be belittled, because it is fundamental to all scientific progress. The other approach is called "applied research." This is investigation carried on for the direct purpose of solving a problem so that the answer will be useful to someone, whether it is the farmer, the drug company, or the astronaut in his rush to reach the moon.

In any case, research has always been an integral part of the academic program at veterinary colleges. The way problems are tackled is related in some measure to the way in which they are financed. Research is financed in three ways. The earliest source and the steadiest has been state oppropriations voted by legislators for solving special problems. In Florida, for example, tax money from race tracks permitted the state to solve many of its parasite problems. The control of parasites has enabled Florida to become a large cattle producing state and, in turn, to enhance its economic status.

Secondly, probably the greatest recent assistance has come from grants made available through the National Institutes of Health. NIH has been very liberal in their consideration of research in animals. Comparative medicine, as it is called, has provided much of the basic knowledge for the advancement in human medicine, because results from work with animals can be extrapolated and applied to human ailments. An example is the cardiology work being done at the University of Pennsylvania, College of Veterinary Medicine. This heart research station is contributing important data on the problem of heart disease in animals, particularly the horse and dog.

The third form of income is that derived from various charitable grant agencies such as the Cancer Fund. There are also commercial enterprises like the Meat Producers Association, which has been a steady contributor to the support of work designed to improve the quality of meat and to reduce the hazards in shipping animals.

Each veterinary college cares for live animals with specific problems and this provides experience for the student and graduate assistant. The veterinarian in practice is encouraged to associate himself with the nearest veterinary college and to keep abreast of the latest advances by attending short courses and seminars there. The veterinarians, the farmers, and the food processors can all turn to the veterinary college for help in solving problems.

In addition to the eighteen veterinary colleges in the United States, there are thirty land grant universities and colleges that have veterinary science departments which are a part of, and administered by, the college of agriculture in the state. The veterinary department at a land grant college is engaged in teaching and research. One of its primary functions is to care for the college herds and flocks that are maintained for teaching agriculture students. Usually there are only one or two veterinarians in such a department, and they teach courses in anatomy, physiology, sanitation, and disease to these prospective farmers and livestock breeders.

Another function of the department is to maintain a diagnostic laboratory to assist farmers and veterinarians on specific disease problems. In connection with many of these laboratories there is research work designed to meet the needs of animal owners and veterinarians in that state. In Montana, for example, the work done on sheep has gained national and international recognition. At Purdue University the veterinary science department is similarly known for its research in swine diseases. It now has a veterinary school in addition to this excellent graduate training center.

In order to progress in the field of teaching and research, it is essential that a course of graduate study be followed. Most of the veterinary colleges offer advanced training in the five major departments. The program is designed to qualify the candidate for the M.S. or the Ph.D. degree.

Companion to these advanced degrees, and sometimes in lieu of them, is specialty certification. To be certified as a specialist, a candidate must have at least three to five years of intensive training and pass a rigid comprehensive examination. The following Specialty Boards in veterinary medicine are recognized by the American Veterinary Medical Association:

- American Board of Veterinary Public Health
- American Board of Veterinary Toxicology
- American College of Laboratory Animal Medicine
- American College of Theriogenologists
- American College of Veterinary Anesthesiologists
- American College of Veterinary Internal Medicine
- American College of Veterinary Microbiologists
- American College of Veterinary Ophthalmologists
- American College of Veterinary Pathologists
- American College of Veterinary Preventive Medicine
- American College of Veterinary Radiology
- American College of Veterinary Surgeons

Certification in the specialty of Public Health indicates that the veterinarian is a specialist in bacterial and viral diseases and outbreaks of sickness they cause. These include such diseases as rabies, hog cholera, anthrax, tuberculosis and brucellosis, all diseases that endanger the health of man, animals and birds.

The veterinary toxicologist deals with the effects of poisons on animals, birds and marine life. These include toxic emissions of smoke, gases and liquids and the toxic effects of insecticides and fertilizers.

Veterinarians who study laboratory animal medicine equip themselves to become members of research teams at hospitals and medical centers. It is difficult to comprehend the growth of the numbers and size of laboratory animal colonies. A quotation from the Humphrey report of 1961 gives some idea of the scope of this field.

The number of animals used in research is increasing each year. It is estimated that 25 million animals: 9 million rats, 900,000 guinea pigs, 50,000 rabbits, 250,000 monkeys, 250,000 dogs and 100,000 cats are used annually in the United States for research teaching, and testing purposes. In addition, many burros, canaries, hamsters, pigeons and chickens are used. The value of all laboratory animals approximates $250 million.

The disease problems of test animals require continued and forceful research. The difficulties of providing animal stocks free of pathogenic organisms must be solved. Another major problem is to stimulate the interest of research workers in the diseases and nutrition of their laboratory animals.

Veterinarians trained in laboratory animal medicine have an extraordinary task of keeping these animals free from their own spontaneous disease as well as caring for them through the procedures of the experiments. They serve as coadministrators of research and as consultants to the animal colonies.

Theriogenologist is a new word to many. Therio means animal form and genology is the knowledge of reproduction. Veterinarians in this field deal with problems of animal reproduction.

The objectives of the veterinary anesthesiologists are to

develop and maintain high standards of anesthesiology for all creatures which include insects, birds, marine life, reptiles and mammals, large and small.

The diplomates of internal medicine are concerned with increasing the competency of those who practice in the field of veterinary internal medicine. These include the subspecialties of cardiology, demnatology, internal medicine and neurology.

Veterinary microbiologists wish to further knowledge and competency in infectious diseases of animals caused by bacteria, mycelia, and viruses. The specialty emphasizes etiology, pathogenesis, transmission immunity, diagnosis, prevention and control.

The veterinary ophthalmologist deals with the eye and sight of all species of animals.

The veterinary pathologist works with his microscope to study disease changes in the cells of the organs. Probably the greatest challenge for the veterinary pathologist is the testing of new drugs which are first tried out on animals. The tissues of each animal receiving the drug is examined for any undesirable changes. Training for this specialty takes five years.

Veterinary preventive medicine deals with the restrictions of the movement of animals from area to area in order to prevent the spread of infectious diseases. This deals with the intra and interstate movement of animals as well as importation and exportation of animals, birds, marine life and insects.

Training in radiology is available at all of the veterinary schools and at a number of human hospitals and medical schools. This field has to do with the use of X-ray and includes taking X-ray pictures as well as the treatment of tumors by radiation and the handling of radioactive compounds. The most useful field is the interpretation of X-ray pictures.

Recent developments in surgery have shown the need for veterinarians with unusual skills in this field. Long difficult procedures are performed on all species.

CHAPTER VIII

Veterinarians in the Armed Forces and Space Medicine

In military service, the veterinary student, like all medical and dental students, finds himself with a privileged status. The ruling on doctors, passed a few years ago, declared members of the three professions essential to the military effort. At that time, veterinarians are allowed to enter the service with the rank of captain. Their military obligation is to serve for two years, most of which is spent in some kind of advanced training in food inspection services, pathology, microbiology, radiobiology, space medicine, or animal care. Many of these jobs are so instructive and interesting that frequently veterinarians decide to make this their career. With its opportunities for study and worldwide travel for a man and his family, such a career is an attractive one.

The salary scale in the armed forces is average or above. The opportunities for training and advancement are exceptional; fringe benefits include medical service for the officer and his family as well as commissary and PX privileges and incentive pay, all of which help reduce living expenses.

Retirement at the end of twenty years is accompanied by one-half regular pay for life. Moreover, the veterinary officer at retirement is usually young enough to enjoy a second career in one of the various other fields of veterinary medicine.

In bridge table conversation it is not unusual to hear something like this, "What, veterinarians in the Army! They dispensed with horses years ago so what could there possibly be for the veterinarian to do?" Even in World War I, when victory on the field depended to a great extent upon horses of the cavalry and artillery, caring for the horses accounted for less than half of the activities of the Veterinary Corps in the Army. The major concern of the veterinarians in military service has always been that of providing safe, edible, nutritious food for the soldiers. Besides food procurement, their work has been expanded to include the preservation of the health of all laboratory and other militarily owned animals which now number in the millions.

One phase of veterinary activity that has been developed as an outgrowth of the K-9 Corps work with dogs in World War II is the procurement, training, and maintenance of hundreds of sentry dogs. These animals have proved their worth in performing as guard dogs at military outposts throughout the world.

At first, veterinarians were civilians employed on a contract basis to treat cavalry and artillery horses. In the Quartermaster's Department they assisted in the purchase of food, particularly meat and dairy products, and were responsible for its wholesomeness. Veterinary assistance in food buying was on a fairly restricted basis until the Spanish American War. In that war it was a tragedy that more soldiers died of dysentery and food poisoning than from

Spanish bullets. In 1916, the Army Veterinary Corps was established in order to insure the services of veterinarians now deemed essential for the health of the troops as well as for animal care. Since that time, the duty of food purchase has comprised over 50 per cent of the work of Army veterinarians.

World War II was the most active time for the Army Veterinary Corps. It was expanded to a strength of 2,200 officers and 5,000 enlisted men. Their main duties at that time were food inspection, environmental health, and research development. Procurement of wholesome nutritious food for the large number of personnel in the military establishments throughout the world required extreme diligence to prevent food-borne disease. The Corps, although it contained over 10 per cent of the veterinarians in America, was small compared to the large number of troops under the colors. The Corps performed a valuable service in protecting the troops from infectious disease and food poisoning during World War II by preventing the contamination of food and water.

As fascinating to hear as any war stories are those told by the veterinarians who went ahead of our men through Italy, bartering for food for our soldiers as they advanced and testing the water to see whether it was safe. Others were responsible for such shipments as a boat load of 450 mules sent to the Eastern Front for work in Burma. During the early occupation of Germany, our veterinarians provided German farmers with vaccines to combat hog cholera in order that production might be increased to meet our needs as well as their own.

Following the war, the Air Force organized its new medical service and established the Air Force Veterinary Corps along with medical and other related corps. The number of veterinary officers has increased with the expanding Air Force to meet new requirements in public health, food inspection, and research. More recently, under the Department of Defense, the Army and Air Force Veterinary Corps are utilized to purchase all food products for the Navy and Marine Corps.

Food inspection by the military veterinary services includes purchasing and contracting for foods, checking cold and dry storage of food supplies, contacting the food industries to have supplies available, improving dehydrated rations, and training and supervising personnel responsible for food inspection. This service-wide food inspection extends to all U.S. military installations at home and abroad. The food is examined with regard to type, class, grade, and specifications. The Army maintains a school in Chicago where it trains both veterinarians and enlisted men of the Veterinary Corps in the grading of eggs and meats, in ordering such items as a carload of hams by Army specifications, and in inspecting and storing perishable foods. This is considered essential for protecting the health of the soldier and the financial interests of the government.

Probably the most interesting and challenging opportunities for veterinarians in the armed forces are in the Division of Research and Development. Assignments are offered in six areas: laboratory animal medicine, pathology, radiology, surgery, virology, and preventive medicine. All of these six areas of medical research and development are of tremendous importance to our future and to our opportunities in the Space Age.

Laboratory animal medicine as a support function in medical research has been developed by military veterinarians to the point where excellent facilities, proper sanitation, humane methods, and disease prevention programs are exemplary. There has also been a Registry of Veterinary Pathology established at the Armed Forces Institute of Pathology as well as a residency program for graduate training in pathology.

Experimental animals also help pave the way for our exploration of outer space. The mouse, the hamster, the rat, the monkey and chimp, the bear, and the donkey are animals now taking a prominent part in our attempt to harness outer space. The achievements of the chimpanzees, Ham and Enos, are familiar to all of us. Their success was made possible by the endless hours of work, experimentation, and development that went into making theirs a safe trip. Animals have been the pioneers who insured the safety of man in later flights. All safety devices are first tried out on animals before they are tried on man. Recently, the bear has proved to be a useful animal in testing safety devices and seat arrangements for aircraft. The space suits and helmets now worn by astronauts were tailored first to fit animals. In all of this, the veterinary officer has had a prominent part in such activities as procuring the animals, perfecting living conditions and building equipment for them, training them, and finally monitoring them through their flights.

You may not have heard of geographic medicine or the armed forces' concern with it. This is the study of health conditions and diseases that would be encountered by American troops if they were called in for military action in a foreign country. As far as possible, all of these conditions are anticipated and studied; this includes testing diets of native food, using concentrated rations, and making up diets for soldiers from native vegetables. Again, animals are used for many testing projects. All the local diseases of a foreign land are studied, including such weird bacterial infections as leprosy and unfamiliar parasitic and virological diseases.

Thus, we see that to maintain our military preparedness in peacetime as well as in times of war, veterinarians must be an integral part of the armed forces.

CHAPTER IX

Veterinarians in Commercial Enterprises

Each year an increasing number of veterinarians are employed in commercial enterprises involving animals. Veterinary supply houses provided the commercial opportunities for veterinarians. Such veterinary establishments cropped up on the East Coast around Boston, New York, and Philadelphia, and in the Midwest in Chicago, Kansas City, and some towns in Iowa.

By 1920, hog cholera serum plants began producing serum and vaccines for hogs. Most of these establishments were small independent businesses that began to appear throughout the Midwest in the cornbelt area where hogs were raised and fattened; there may have been as many as fifty or sixty of these. It was not long before the more successful serum companies began buying out the less active ones as well as taking over some of the early Eastern firms. Gradually many of these companies merged until there were eight or ten supplying the profession.

Many veterinarians were employed to sell serum and vaccine, as well as drugs, instruments, and other biological products to the practitioners. Assisting the salesman in each firm was a serviceman or trouble shooter. This veterinarian, trained in bacteriology and pathology, specialized in animal diseases, usually swine diseases. Veterinarians were also employed as production men for the plants, while others did research pertaining to new products that they were developing.

Concurrent with this, pharmaceutical companies producing medicine for humans also developed. These were much larger and dealt in far greater volume of business. Following World War II, it was found that many drug products were useful for both man and animals; therefore, to increase their volume of sales, the pharmaceutical companies began to develop veterinary divisions. Then the large pharmaceutical houses proceeded to buy up the smaller serum companies until today each of the old veterinary supply houses and serum companies is a part of some large drug corporation.

With the advantage of national and international advertising and distribution, the field has grown and there are increasing opportunities for veterinarians in sales promotion, service, and production. Veterinarians are also in demand to do research on product development and to conduct toxicity and control tests to see that drugs, vaccines, and all pharmaceutical products are suitable and safe for human and animal consumption.

Animals, mostly rats, monkeys and dogs, are used for toxicity tests. Tissues of laboratory animals receiving the products must be examined to see whether a specific drug causes degeneration of any of the organs of the animals. As the compounds used become more complex, so does the problem of testing for toxicity. Veterinarians doing this work have to be well trained in the field of pathology in order to make proper interpretations. They are in great demand and earn from $18,000 to $50,000 annually.

Animal foods manufactured for and distributed to livestock owners amount to a multi-billion-dollar operation each year. Of this, 400 million dollars is dog food alone. The production of both animal and human food in recent years has become more complicated because much manufactured food is supplemented with minerals and vitamins. For example, all special infant diets and supplemental food for babies must be tested on animals and assayed before being put on the market.

Similarly, in animal feeds, to take one instance, the addition of antibiotics to swine rations promotes rapid growth because it eliminates minor infections. Assaying must be supervised by someone familiar with animals, and veterinarians are best suited for this work. The testing and supervision of feed manufacturing requires a number of specially trained veterinarians, who are well compensated for service in this field.

We have already touched on the veterinarian's role as government meat inspectors. Another pertinent field in the meat-packing industry is by-products. For example, drugs such as insulin, pituitary extracts, and ACTH are produced from the extracts of the endocrine glands. Satisfying professional achievement of a high order is to be found here.

Raising laboratory animals to meet the demands of the recent rapid development of animal research has opened a new field. The breeding and growing of healthy laboratory animals for research institutions is now a flourishing enterprise. The production of germ-free animals is a highly scientific process for which well-trained veterinary talent is needed. As indicated in Chapter VII, millions of mice and rats and hundreds of thousands of rabbits, guinea pigs, cats, dogs, and monkeys must be raised annually to meet the demands of research laboratories.

The veterinary publishing business is another very interesting field. The publication of scientific books of a veterinary nature, as well as the monthly and semi-monthly scientific journals and special material for promotion of veterinary products, offers employment to a limited number of veterinarians. There are probably no more than fifty men so engaged at the present time, but those interested in journalism will do well to look into this field.

CHAPTER X

Veterinarians in Nutrition

Veterinary nutrition is one of the most important, and yet one of the newer and least developed, areas in veterinary medicine. This specialty has excellent potential for the young graduate who wants to take some graduate training. The advanced training should be in biochemistry, physiology, nutritional requirements of animals, pathology, and genetics.

The veterinary nutritionist's most important function is as special adviser to the livestock owner. Success for the livestockman today depends upon getting the animals to a marketable age in the shortest amount of time with the least amount of food. Hence, the veterinarian's value is an economic one based upon his ability to increase the stockman's profits.

In such a position, the veterinarian's first problem is to prevent contamination of the feed lots. Feed lot facilities, as far as equipment is concerned, are expensive and cannot be moved to new areas but have to be used over and over again. It is not uncommon for animals newly admitted to the feed lot to become sick with either respiratory or digestive ailments. These diseases, many of which are chronic, slow down growth and development, and lengthen the fattening period. Parasites, both internal and external, also infest the animals and cause disease. All of these delays in fattening are figured in terms of added dollars to the cost of the operation.

Drugs, both antibiotics and parasiticides, have been added to feed to control bacterial diseases and parasites. Preparing formulas for feed, which will keep animals in good condition during the growing and fattening period, is a job for a well-trained scientist. In addition to the disease prohibitors, many additive compounds have been tried to hasten the growth, development, and finishing of animals for the market; additional new ones are being considered every day and there are undoubtedly many more that will soon be discovered.

The veterinarian is also needed as a consultant and adviser to feed companies. One of the problems in such a position would be the search for toxic substances in feeds. Certain weeds and weed seeds are toxic and cause death to large numbers of animals. The feed manufacturer needs advice in selecting the ingredients for compounding feed for animals so that they will not lose weight or become ill and die.

In the commercial feed business, selecting ingredients for feeds takes experience and good training, and the problems are constantly changing. Some years certain cereals and grains are plentiful and low in price when others are scarce and expensive. Feed formulas must be adjusted accordingly to save money. For example, use of ground corn cobs for roughage has proved to be profitable in a year when hay is scarce. It is the nutritionist's job to see that rations are balanced and that the animals make maximum gains and fatten quickly.

Genetics is another consideration in raising livestock profitably. Certain strains of animals may have lethal genetic factors that make the animals unprofitable to raise, while other strains breed and grow rapidly. Consultation with a trained veterinarian may avert trouble in a flock or herd.

Often when an old feed lot is used, the raising and feeding of sheep and swine may become almost impossible because of infections. In these instances, the infected lots have to be "rested" and new lots acquired. Nowadays, new pastures and feed lots are often stocked with what is known as disease-free animals.

In order to produce disease-free animals, healthy pregnant mothers are operated on at term by Caesarian section and the young are taken and raised by specially prepared formula under sterile conditions. The young orphan is kept warm in an incubator until it gains enough maturity to shift for itself and eat regular food. Then it is taken to new pastures and lots that have been made disease free. These animals are raised and fattened for market or used for future breeding stock. This method provides the producer with new healthy animals for his farm. Veterinarians are needed to supervise and direct these disease-free establishments.

In producing race horses, both thoroughbreds and standard breds, the breeders and trainers are out to produce specimens that will mature rapidly enough to win at the tracks at an early age and be durable enough to continue racing for a long period of time. The successful racing career of a horse depends on a suitable diet and healthy body. The owners need advice for improving nutrition and disease control. In race horses parasites are also a problem. Drugs added to the ration, as well as rotation of pastures, have done much to keep these animals free of parasites.

Special diets are needed for dogs, especially for the young growing pup. Intestinal ailments are common in pups, and commercial prescription diets are available to correct these. More such diets are being developed to meet other special conditions.

It is not uncommon to find kidney ailments in the middle-aged and old dog. Restoring the health of these dogs depends to a large extent on nutrition. Diets of a special protein can help to keep kidneys functioning. The nutritionist must analyze deficiencies and adjust the diet accordingly.

The veterinary nutritionist has a very definite place in veterinary medicine and as time goes on there will be greater need for people to be so trained. Remuneration is good and in line with the salaries quoted in other fields of the profession.

CHAPTER XI

Opportunities in Veterinary Science

Marine Biology, Oceanography and the Veterinarian

You may think that the ships and the fishing boats are as remote from veterinary medicine as another planet. But below the ocean's surface there is a multitude of living things darting, watching, living and dying and this continuation of life tests the imagination and curiosity of all those who care about living things, including the veterinarian. The oceans have fascinated man since the days of his earliest ventures into new worlds. Exploring its depths offers the veterinarian a new professional role.

Over the past 35 years there has been an exciting increase in the understanding of what lives below the sometimes calm and other times turmoil of the ocean surface. There has been an ever increasing interest brought about by a variety of new instruments and methods which gives access to greater and greater depths. The resources of animal life in the sea await development to assist with the ever mounting task of keeping man from starving.

The animals of the sea present an incredible diversity with 200,000 species already identified and many new ones being found on every new oceanographic expedition. The annual income to the world's fishermen from marine catches is now roughly $8 billion. The prospects are that the ocean can be cultivated and harvested more intensively and in a greater variety of ways than ever before. In order to husband these resources and use them wisely the Marine Biologist with a background in veterinary medicine could play a prominent role in this development.

These few remarks should point up the need for scientific research and development to enhance the future use of sea animals as a source of food to save the world from starving. The need of the veterinarians with learning in marine biology, husbandry and oceanography is self evident and this new and exciting field offers a great challenge to those who prepare for it.

Alternate Career Opportunities

This book deals with a career in veterinary medicine, but for some of you who have studied the contents, becoming a veterinarian may be beyond your reach in terms of time, effort and financial backing. If so, and if your heart is set on working with animals, consider the opportunities in a new field, that of "Laboratory Animal Science."

Just as the physician and dentist need medical and dental assistants to make up the team that offer health service, so does the research veterinarian need trained assistants.

Laboratory animal science is a fairly recent field in which special skills and competence are necessary in order to care for and handle animals in the daily practice of veterinary medicine research as well as in teaching. The research and teaching team "laboratory animal scientist" may include the breeder of animals as well as the user, but the title, as used here, means a person trained to assist legally professional personnel such as veterinarians, physiologists, microbiologists, physicians and dentists in animal research. The field offers good opportunities to both men and women.

Workers in this field are employed by medical, veterinary and dental schools, hospitals, research and teaching institutions, pharmaceutical houses, breeders of laboratory animals and as assistants to veterinarians. They may work in the food and drug industries, in fish and wildlife services and in many other diversified technical programs carried on by the state and federal governments.

High school preparation for such training should include four years of English, two to four years of mathematics, one year of chemistry, one year of physics and one year of biology.

Training for a career in laboratory animal science presently exists at a number of colleges and universities in widely scattered areas in this country. The curriculum extends over a period of two years and leads to a diploma as an Associate in Arts and Applied Science. In those instances where students are stimulated to continue their undergraduate collegiate education they may do so and receive the bachelor's degree. The salary levels offered for such employment are on a level with those of similarly trained laboratory workers.

Accredited Programs in Animal Technology

Alabama
* Snead State Junior College
  Animal Hospital Technology
  Program
  Boaz, AL 35957

California
  Los Angeles Pierce College
  Animal Health Technology
  Program
  6201 Winnetka Avenue
  Woodland Hills, CA 92101
  Cosumnes River College
  Animal Health Technology
  Program
  8401 Center Parkway
  Sacramento, CA 95823
* Foothill de Anza Community College
  Animal Health Technician
  Program
  12345 El Monte Road
  Los Altos Hills, CA 94022
* Mt. San Antonio College
  Animal Health Technology
  Program
  1100 North Grand Avenue
  Walnut, CA 91789
* Orange Coast College
  Animal Health Technology
  Program
  2701 Fairview Road
  Costa Mesa, CA 92626
* San Diego Mesa College
  Animal Health Technology
  Program
  7250 Mesa College Drive
  San Diego, CA 92111
* Yuba College
  Animal Health Technician
  Program
  Beale Road and Linda Avenue
  Marysville, CA 95901

Colorado
  Colorado Mountain College
  Animal Health Technology
  Program
  West Campus
  Glenwood Springs, CO 81601
  Bel-Rea Institute of Animal Technology
  9870 East Alameda
  Denver, CO 80231

Connecticut
* Quinnipiac College
  Laboratory Animal Technology
  Mt. Carmel Avenue
  Hamden, CT 06518

Florida
  St. Petersburg Junior College
  Veterinary Technology
  Program
  St. Petersburg, FL 33733

Georgia
  Abraham Baldwin Agriculture College
  Animal Health Technology
  Program
  Box 8, ABAC Station
  Tifton, GA 31794

* Probational Accreditation

* Fort Valley State College
  Animal Health Technology
    Program
  Fort Valley, GA 31030
Illinois
  Parkland College
  Veterinary Technology
    Program
  2400 Bradley
  Champaign, IL 61820
Indiana
  Purdue University
  School of Veterinary Medicine
  Veterinary Technology
    Program
  West Lafayette, IN 47907
Kansas
  Colby Community College
  Animal Technology Program
  1255 South Range
  Colby, KS 67701
Kentucky
  Morehead State University
  Veterinary Technology
    Program
  Box 702
  Morehead, KY 40351
Maine
* Dept. of Animal & Veterinary
    Sciences
  Animal Medical Technology
    Program
  University of Maine
  Orono, ME 04473
Maryland
* Essex Community College
  Animal Science Technician
    Program
  7201 Rossville Blvd.
  Baltimore, MD 21237
* Garrett Community College
  Veterinary Technology
    Program
  McHenry, MD 21541
Massachusetts
* Newberry Junior College
  Holliston Campus
  921 Boylston St.
  Boston, MA 02115
* Becker Junior College
  Veterinary Assistant Program
  1003 Old Main Street
  Leicester, MA 01524
Michigan
  Wayne County Community
    College
  Animal Health Technician
    Training Program
  540 E. Canfield
  Detroit, MI 48201
  Michigan State University
  College of Veterinary Medicine
  Animal Technology Program
  East Lansing, MI 48823
* Macomb County Community
    College
  Veterinary Technician
    Program
  Center Campus
  P.O. Box 309
  Warren, MI 48093
Minnesota
  University of Minnesota
  Animal Health Technology
    Program
  Waseca, MN 56093

Missouri
Maple Woods Community College
Animal Health Technology Program
2601 N.E. Barry Road
Kansas City, MO 64156
Northeast Missouri State University
Animal Health Technology Program
Kirksville, MO 63501
* Jefferson College
Animal Health Technology Program
Hillsboro, MO 63050

Nebraska
University of Nebraska
School of Technical Agriculture
Veterinary Technology Program
Curtis, NE 69025

New Jersey
Camden County College
Animal Science Technology Program
P.O. Box 200
Blackwood, NJ 08012

New York
* State University of New York
Agricultural & Technical College
Veterinary Science Technology Dept.
Delhi, NY 13753
State University of New York
Agricultural & Technical College
Agriculture and Life Sciences
Canton, NY 13617

North Carolina
Central Carolina Technical Institute
Veterinary Medical Technology Program
1105 Kelly Drive
Sanford, NC 27330

North Dakota
North Dakota State University
Animal Health Technician Program
Department of Veterinary Science
Fargo, ND 58102

Ohio
Columbus Technical Institute
Animal Health Technology Program
550 East Springs Street
Columbus, OH 43215
Raymond Walters College
Animal Health Technology Program
University of Cincinnati
Cincinnati, OH 45221

Pennsylvania
Harcum Junior College
Animal Technician Program
Bryn Mawr, PA 19010

South Carolina
Tri-County Technical College
Animal Health Technology Program

P.O. Box 587
Pendleton, SC 29670

Tennessee
Columbia State Community College
Animal Health Technology Program
Columbia, TN 38401

Texas
* Texas State Technical Institute
Animal Medical Technology Program
James Connally Campus
Waco, TX 76705
Frank Phillips College
Animal Health Technology Program
Box 311
Borger, TX 79007
Sul Ross State University
Range Animal Science Department
Animal Technology Program
Alpine, TX 78839
* Cedar Valley College
Animal Medical Technology Program
3030 N. Dallas Ave.
Lancaster, TX 75134

Virginia
Blue Ridge Community College
Animal Technology Program
Box 80
Weyers Cave, VA 24486
* Northern Virginia Community College
Animal Science Technology Program
Loudoun Campus
1000 Harry Flood Byrd Highway
Sterling, VA 22170

Washington
Fort Stellacoom Community College
Animal Technology Program
9401 Farwest Dr., S.W.
Tacoma, WA 98498

Wisconsin
*Madison Area Technical College.
Animal Technician Program
211 North Carroll Street
Madison, WI 53703

Wyoming
- Eastern Wyoming College
Animal Health Technology Program
3200 West C Street
Torrington, WY 82240

* Probational Accreditation

CHAPTER XII

Women in Veterinary Medicine

Women are welcomed and needed in the profession of veterinary medicine. You will probably be surprised by the outstanding role they are playing today in this field. All the schools of America and most of the world accept women on a non-discrimatory basis. For example, the University of Pennsylvania has accepted as many as 50 per cent women in some classes in recent years. This large number is not surprising because the applications for admission from women run about this percentage and there is no difference between the academic records, experiences and motivation of the two sexes.

The female graduates are actively engaged in all branches of veterinary medicine in about the same proportion as are men. The highest percentage of them are engaged in practice working with both large and small animals. For some reason never explained, equine practice has an unusual appeal for women. Besides practice they are engaged in teaching, research, public health, poultry and meat inspection, care of laboratory animals, pathology, zoo work, drug testing, wild life, marine life and the armed forces.

CHAPTER XIII

The Veterinarian's License to Practice and the Code of Ethics

The well-trained and honest professional person can be relied upon to render good service to the community. However, there are always some charlatans who endeavor to imitate these reputable people and thus subject the general public to substandard and fraudulent practices. Occasionally livestock owners are approached by those who pose as veterinarians and who offer their services in treating livestock. These people may try to sell hog feed, remedies for lameness in race horses, or cures for breeding ailments in cattle. Proprietors of pet shops have been known to pretend to be veterinarians, examine dogs, treat them with parasiticides and other remedies, and even vaccinate them. Each state has laws designed to protect the owners of both large and pet animals from these untrained individuals, and all veterinary doctors must be licensed.

In order to obtain a license, a person must have a degree from an accredited veterinary college, must be a United States citizen of good character, and must pass a qualifying examination in the state in which he wants to practice.

Occasionally a state reviews an application from someone who has been educated in a veterinary school outside the United States. There are two Canadian schools, both of which have been approved, and if a graduate signifies his intent to become a citizen of the United States he is eligible to take the examination for licensing. Some schools in England and other countries have been similarly approved. Graduates of some of the veterinary schools in South America, Europe, and the Far East present more difficult problems when it comes to making a judgment on whether they are eligible to take examinations. The schools in some of these regions are on the approved list, while others are not. In any event, a foreign candidate wishing to acquire a license should first be able to communicate fluently in English, he should be familiar with the problems and customs of the state in which he wishes to practice, and he should have signified his intentions to become a citizen of this country by taking out his first papers.

A few years ago, through our national association, the American Veterinary Medical Association, the National Board of Veterinary Examiners was established. Their comprehensive examination on all subjects of veterinary medicine has been made available to the examining boards of each state so that the knowledge of the veterinarian applying for a license can be tested. The majority of states now use the national board questions, and, in addition, each state has its own specific requirements. The problems in a state such as Florida are peculiar to it because climate, vegetation, livestock, and disease vary greatly from the state of Minnesota, for example. It is for this reason that very few states have reciprocity with one another. Veterinarians must prepare themselves in order to be judged competent by the state in which they want to practice. The veterinarian moving to another state is required to pass the examination of that state before he is allowed to practice.

Most licenses must be renewed on a yearly basis to keep them active. A nominal fee is usually charged for annual renewal. Prosecution for a major offense in most states renders the license void. That is, if a person is found guilty of a crime and sentenced to serve in a penitentiary, his license is automatically suspended. In addition to the state license, it is required that each veterinarian examining and approving animals for interstate and international shipment be approved and licensed by the federal government.

Veterinarians, like physicians, take an oath at the time they enter the profession.

The Veterinarian's Oath

"Being admitted to the profession of veterinary medicine, I solemnly dedicate myself and the knowledge I possess to the benefit of society, to the conservation of our livestock resources, and to the relief of suffering to animals. I will practice my profession conscientiously with dignity. The health of my patients, the best interest of their owners, and the welfare of my fellow man, will be my primary consideration.

"I will, at all times, be humane and temper pain with anesthesia where indicated. I will not use my knowledge contrary to the laws of humanity, nor in contravention to the ethical code of my profession. I will uphold and strive to advance the honor and noble traditions of the veterinary profession.

"These pledges I make freely in the eyes of God and upon my honor."

To further implement this oath, veterinarians are guided by the "Principles of Veterinary Medical Ethics" prepared by the American Veterinary Medical Association Judicial Council, which has surveillance over the professional conduct of veterinarians. In it are set forth the standards in such matters as advertising, professional responsibilities, listing in telephone directories, professional cards, merchandising, drug display, emergency service, endorsement of remedies and cures, and general conduct of the professional person.

The Rotary International Service Club, to which many veterinarians belong, has a Four-Way test, based on the Golden Rule, which is a good guide in problems of conduct and ethics. An individual can determine whether his decision in dealing with a problem is an honorable one by asking himself four questions:

1. Is it the TRUTH?
2. Is it FAIR to all concerned?
3. Will it build GOODWILL and BETTER FRIENDSHIPS?
4. Will it be BENEFICIAL to all concerned?

If the answer is unequivocally "yes" in each instance, then he may rest assured that his decision is an ethical one. If his answer is "perhaps" or "I don't know," the chances are that the situation should be studied further.

All professional associations have as one purpose the attainment of better ethical standards. When men become better acquainted, they are able to discuss and exchange views as they work coöperatively under an agreed code of conduct.

CHAPTER XIV

Your Future in Veterinary Medicine

In summary, may I reaffirm my conviction that veterinary medicine offers a way of life rich in opportunity. Although it requires, as do all the professions, a serious and prolonged preparation, the rewards are considerable. These include the satisfaction of being of real service in this life both to animals and man, the stimulation of intellectual achievement inherent in keeping abreast of the field as it advances, the prestige accorded to the professional man because it is understood that he fulfills an important function in community life, and the compensation of a good income in accordance with one's efforts.

One other great advantage in these days of inevitable regimentation in huge corporations and government structures is that this is one of the few remaining careers that allows you to be independent in choosing your own location and gearing your work to suit your pace. More than that, your services are always needed.

In veterinary medicine, as in human medicine, most doctors aspire, by and large, to treat patients. But many other avenues are open, and, as indicated in each chapter, the opportunities in all of these fields are increasing. Not only is there plenty of work to do here at home, but, as pointed out, in order for the human race to survive we must increase food supplies abroad, too. Animal protein, which is so essential, is relatively even more scarce than grains. There is bold adventure awaiting those who have the vision and vitality to pioneer in solving the problems of how to raise, protect, and distribute enough animals to provide this food. Controlling disease and increasing production are areas in which the veterinarian can do great service.

The American Veterinary Medical Association has a great interest in young people who are considering veterinary medicine as a career. You may write them for literature and any questions you ask will be given courteous and thoughtful attention.

APPENDIX I

College of Veterinary Medicine in the United States

Auburn University, School of Veterinary Medicine, Auburn, AL 36849, Dr. J. T. Vaughan, Dean.
University of California, School of Veterinary Medicine, Davis, CA 95616, Dr. William R. Prichard, Dean.
Colorado State University, College of Veterinary Medicine and Biomedical Sciences, Ft. Collins, CO 80523, Dr. Robert D. Phemister, Dean.
Cornell University, New York State College of Veterinary Medicine. Ithaca, NY 14853, Dr. Edward C. Melby, Jr., Dean.
University of Florida, College of Veterinary Medicine, Gainesville, FL 32610, Dr. Kirk N. Gelett, Dean.
University of Georgia, College of Veterinary Medicine, Athens, GA 30602, Dr. David P. Anderson, Dean.
University of Illinois, College of Veterinary Medicine, Urbana, IL 61801, Dr. R. E. Dierks, Dean.
Iowa State University, College of Veterinary Medicine, Ames, IA 50011, Dr. Phillip T. Pearson, Dean.

Kansas State University, College of Veterinary Medicine, Manhattan, KS 66502, Dr. D. M. Trotter, Dean.

Louisiana State University, School of Veterinary Medicine, Baton Rouge, LA 70803, Dr. Evertt D. Besch, Dean.

Michigan State University, College of Veterinary Medicine, East Lansing, MI 48824, Dr. John R. Weiser, Dean.

University of Minnesota, College of Veterinary Medicine, St. Paul, MN 55103, Dr. R. H. Dunlop, Dean.

Mississippi State University, College of Veterinary Medicine, Mississippi State, MS 39762, Dr. James Miller, Dean.

University of Missouri, College of Veterinary Medicine, Columbia, MO 65211, Dr. Kenneth D. Weide, Dean.

North Carolina State University, School of Veterinary Medicine, Raleigh, NC 27650.

Ohio State University, College of Veterinary Medicine, Columbus, OH 43210, Dr. Ronald A. Wright, Dean.

Oklahoma State University, College of Veterinary Medicine, Stillwater, OK 74074, Dr. Patrick Morgan, Dean.

Oregan State University, School of Veterinary Medicine, Corvallis, OR 97331, Dr. E. E. Wedman, Dean.

University of Pennsylvania, School of Veterinary Medicine, Philadelphia, PA 19104, Dr. Robert R. Marshak, Dean.

Purdue University, School of Veterinary Medicine, West Lafayette, IN 47907, Dr. Jack J. Stockton, Dean.

University of Tennessee, College of Veterinary Medicine, Knoxville, TN 39701, Dr. Hyram Kitchen, Dean.

Texas A & M University, College of Veterinary Medicine, College Station, TX 77843, Dr. George C. Shelton, Dean.

Tufts University, School of Veterinary Medicine, Boston, MA 02111, Dr. W. Robert Cook, acting Dean.

Tuskegee Institute, School of Veterinary Medicine, Tuskegee Institute, AL 36088, Dr. Walter C. Bowie, Dean.

Virginia Tech and University of Maryland, Virginia-Maryland Regional College of Veterinary Medicine, Blacksburg, VA 24061, Dr. Richard B. Talbot, Dean.

Washington State University, College of Veterinary Medicine, Pullman, WA 99163, Dr. Leo K. Bustad, Dean.

University of Wisconsin, School of Veterinary Medicine, Madison, WI 53706, Dr. Bernard C. Easterday, Dean.

APPENDIX II

Veterinary Associations

American Veterinary Medical Association
930 N. Meacham Road
Schaumburg, Illinois   60172
Dr. D. A. Price, Executive Vice-President

Canadian Veterinary Medical Association
360 Bronson Ave., Ms. Sylvia Burns
Ottawa KIR 6J3, Ontario, Canada

American Animal Hospital Association
3612 E. Jefferson Blvd., Robert M. Hanson
South Bend, Indiana   46660

Women's Veterinary Medical Association
5713 Lone Tree Drive, Dr. Jane Robens
Bethesda, Maryland   20014

American Association of Bovine Practitioners
P. O. Box 2319, Dr. H. E. Amstutz
W. Lafayette, Indiana   47906

American Association of Equine Practitioners
Route 5, 22363 Hillcrest Circle, Dr. W. O. Kester
Golden, Colorado 80401

American Association of Feline Practitioners
3447 Lyndane Ave. S., Dr. Mike McMenomy
Minneapolis, MN 55408

American Association of Sheep and Goat Practitioners
Dr. Don E. Bailey, 248 N.W. Garden Valley
Roseburg, OR 97470

American Association of Swine Practitioners
5921 Fleur Dr., Dr. F. D. Wertman
Des Moines, IA 50321

American Association of Zoo Veterinarians
Dr. Morton J. Silberman, Emory University
Atlanta, GA 30322

American Society of Laboratory Animal Practitioners
Dr. Ronald L. Bell, Sec.-Treas.
Department of Lab. Animals
Ohio State University Hospitals
333 West 10th Ave.
Columbus, Ohio 43210

American College of Laboratory Animal Medicine
Dr. William S. Webster
Depart. of Animal Medicine
University of Massachusetts Medical School
55 Lake Ave., North
Worcester MA 01605

There are many other veterinary associations devoted to particular phases of the profession. However, because their secretaryships change from year to year, it is advisable to direct inquiries to the American Veterinary Medical Association in Chicago.

APPENDIX III

Bibliography

Bierer, B. W. "Short History of Veterinary Medicine in America." East Lansing, Michigan: Michigan State University Press, 1955.

Bridges, W. "Zoo Doctor." New York: Wm. Morrow and Co., Inc., 1957.

De Kruif, Paul Henry. "Hunger Fighters." New York: Harcourt Brace and Co., 1928.

Dinsmore, R. J. " 'Hoss' Doctor." Boston: Waverly House, 1940.

Goldhaft, Arthur D. "The Golden Egg." New York: Horizon Press, 1957.

Greene, Carla. "I Want to be an Animal Doctor." Chicago: Childrens Press (Juvenile), 1956.

Hancock, R. C. G. "Memoirs of a Veterinary Surgeon." London: MacGibbon and Kee, 1952.

Henderson, J. Y., and Taplinger, Richard. "Circus Doctor." Boston: Little, Brown and Co., 1951.

Herriot, James. "All Creatures Great and Small." New York: St. Martin's Press, 1971.

Herriot, James. "All Things Bright and Beautiful." New York: St. Martin's Press, 1973.

———, "The Lord God Made Them All." New York: St. Martin's Press, 1981.

Knott, Middleton Murray. "Gone Away with O'Malley." New York: Doubleday Doran, 1944.

Leckie, Victor C. "A Centaur Looks Back." London: Hodder and Slaughton, 1946.

Moon, G. R. "How to Become a Doctor." New York: McGraw-Hill Book Co., 1950.

Perry, John and Jane G. "Veterinarians and What They Do." New York: Franklin Watts, Inc.

Porter, James A. "Doctor Spare My Cow." Ames, Iowa: Iowa State College Press, 1956.

Roothaert, A. "Dutch Vet." New York: The Macmillan Company, 1940.

Smithcors, J. F. "Evolution of the Veterinary Art." Kansas City, Missouri: Veterinary Medicine Publishing Co., 1957.

U.S. BAI. "Career Opportunities for Graduate Veterinarians in BAI." Washington: Government Printing Office, 1952.

U.S. Senate. "Veterinary Medical Science and Human Health." Washington: Government Printing Office, 1961.

Vine, Louis L. "Dogs in My Life." New York: Appleton-Century Crofts, 1961.

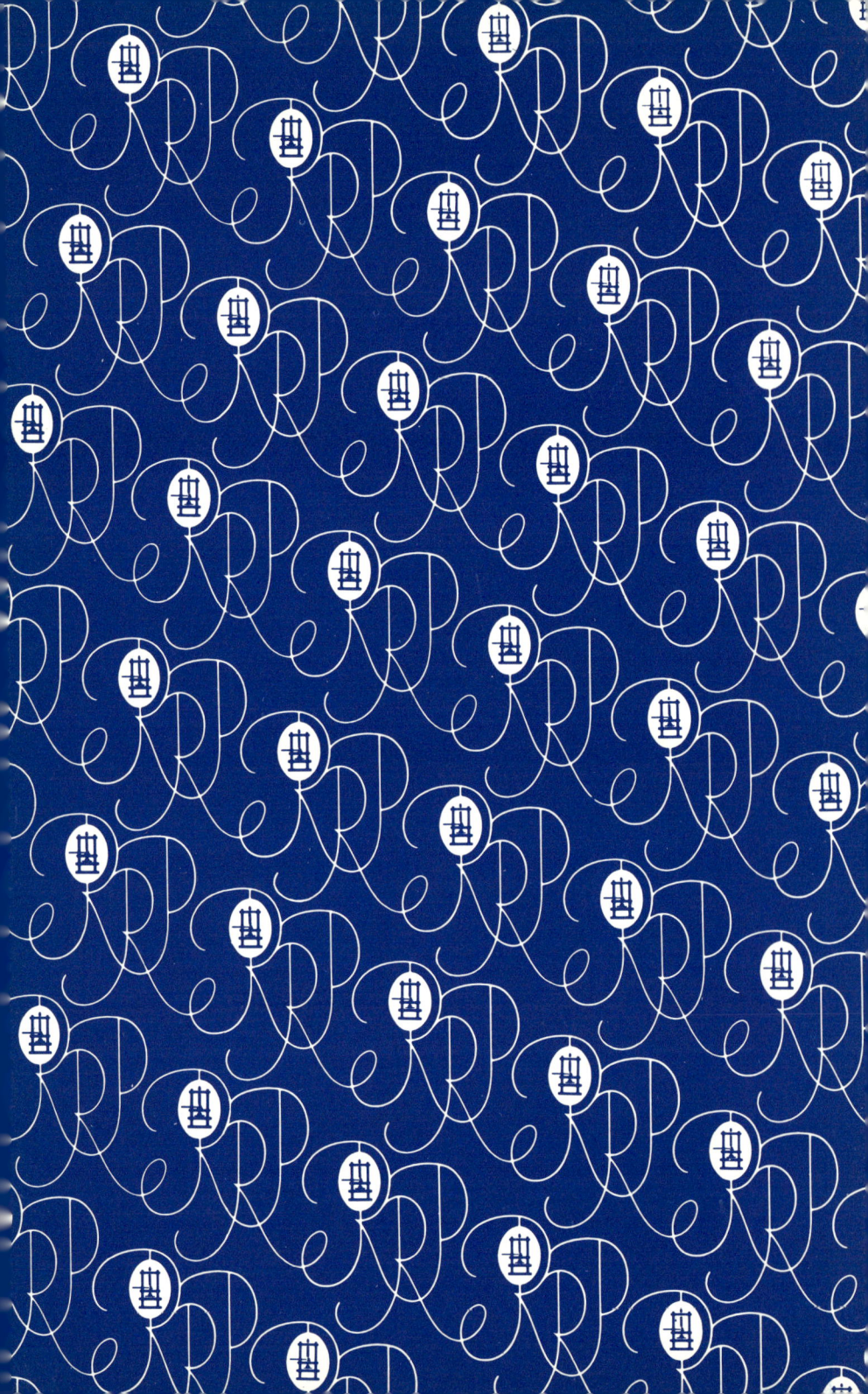